RENAL DIET COOKBOOK

Mix of pineapple and carrots

Ingredients

- 1 packet Knox unflavored gelatin
- 300 ml apricot nectar
- 240g canned crushed pineapple
- 1/2 cup sugar
- 240g low fat cream cheese
- 1 cup heavy whipping cream
- 1 cup shredded carrots

Method

1. Put a glass bowl and beaters of a hand mixer into the freezer to chill.
2. Pour 1 cup of the apricot nectar into a small saucepan and heat to a low boil. Place gelatin in a bowl and pour heated nectar into the gelatin and whisk to dissolve.
3. Pour remaining nectar and canned pineapple, including juice, into the gelatin mixture. Stir in carrots. Place in the refrigerator until partially set.
4. In a separate bowl, combine the cream cheese and sugar. Set aside.
5. Remove chilled glass bowl from the freezer and pour in the heavy whipping cream. Beat on high speed for 3-4 minutes to whip. Gently fold whipped cream into the cream cheese mixture.
6. Pour the cream cheese mixture into the partially set gelatin mixture and blend gently with a whisk or spoon. Refrigerate for 3-4 hours.

Cranberry and marshmallow mix

Ingredients

- 2 and a 1/2 cups fresh cranberries
- 4 medium Red Delicious apples
- 1 tablespoon Fruit-Fresh Produce Protector
- 1/4 cup sugar
- 1 cup miniature marshmallows

Method

1. Peel and core apples. Place apples and cranberries in a food processor and chop.
2. Sprinkle with Fruit-Fresh and mix well.
3. Fold in sugar and marshmallows.
4. Chill at least 4 hours.
5. Stir and serve.

Creamy grapes

Ingredients

- 3 pounds seedless grapes

- 240g low-fat cream cheese
- 240g sour cream
- 1/2 cup sugar
- 2 teaspoons vanilla extract

Method

1. Set cream cheese out to soften.
2. Slice grapes in half vertically.
3. Mix softened cream cheese, sour cream, sugar and vanilla in a medium-sized bowl.
4. Fold in grapes.
5. Chill and serve.

Gelatinous pineapple

Ingredients

- 2 cups cottage cheese
- 90g lime gelatin mix
- 2 cups canned pineapple tidbits (Packed in juice)
- 240g whipped topping

Method

1. In a medium-sized bowl, sprinkle dry gelatin over cottage cheese.
2. In a large bowl, mix whipped topping and drained pineapple together.
3. Fold whipped topping and fruit mixture into cottage cheese mixture. Cover and refrigerate overnight.

Flaky coconut pineapples

Ingredients

- 240g canned crushed pineapple in juice
- 330g canned mandarin oranges
- 1/2 cup mini marshmallows
- 1/4 cup sour cream
- 2 tablespoons flaked coconut
- 8 maraschino cherries

Method

1. Drain pineapple and oranges well.
2. Once drained, mix all other ingredients in a bowl.
3. Chill overnight.

Cheesy veggie salad

Ingredients

- 1 cucumber
- 450g canned low-sodium sliced beets
- 4 teaspoons balsamic vinegar
- 2 teaspoons canola oil
- 2 tablespoons Gorgonzola cheese

Method

1. Thinly slice cucumber.
2. Place beet slices on a serving plate.
3. Layer cucumber slices on top of beet slices.
4. Drizzle with vinegar and oil.
5. Sprinkle with Gorgonzola cheese.

Autumn wild rice

Ingredients

- 2 tablespoons raisins
- 2 cups apples
- ½ cup quick cooking wild rice (Uncooked)
- ¼ cup celery
- ¾ cup carrots
- ¼ cup green bell pepper
- ¼ teaspoon black pepper
- ¼ teaspoon dried whole sage
- 1 and a ½ cups reduced-sodium Vegetable Stock
- ¼ cup fresh lemon juice
- ¾ cup converted rice (Uncooked)
- 1 fresh sage sprig (optional)

Method

1. Take the raisins in a bowl and add ¼ cup hot water. Let the raisins stand in the hot water for about 5 minutes before draining the water completely. Set aside the raisins in the bowl.

2. Read the instructions on the package of wild rice and prepare the quick cooking wild rice. Remove the pan from the heat when done and set it aside as well.

3. Take the celery, apples and bell pepper and chop them up. Take the carrots and shred them.

4. Take a non-stick skillet or a pan and coat it with cooking spray all over. Place it over medium flame and heat it until it has become hot enough. Place the celery, apple, carrot and green pepper into the pan and sauté them until they have become crisp and tender. Take the skillet or pan off the heat and set aside as well.

5. Take another saucepan and add the 1 and a ½ cups of reduced sodium vegetable stock, pepper and sage. Mix them together and bring it to a boil. Add in the converted rice and also give it a stir. Cover the saucepan and heat and simmer it for 20 minutes or until the rice becomes tender and the liquid has been absorbed completely.

6. Take away the saucepan from the heat and add in the raisins, wild rice, apple mixture and also the juice of the lemon. Cover the pan and let it stay like that for 5 minutes.

7. You are ready to serve and place portions of it into a serving bowl. You can garnish it with sage springs, if you want.

Fresh green salad

Ingredients

- 1 carrot (Sliced)
- 4 cups red leaf or other lettuce (Shredded)
- 2 radishes (Sliced)
- 2 cucumbers (Sliced)
- 2 celery stalks (Sliced)
- 1 large bell pepper (Diced or sliced into rings)

Method
1. Take a large bowl and add all the vegetables to it and mix them together.
2. You can serve this with your favourite salad dressing.

Kidney friendly yellow squash

Ingredients

- 2 tablespoons margarine or butter (Melted)
-
$1/8$ teaspoon black pepper

- ¾ teaspoon thyme
- 1 medium onion (Chopped)
- 2 cans yellow squash (Sliced)
- 1 tablespoon lemon juice
- 1 large bell pepper (Chopped)
- 1 small celery stalk (Chopped)

Method

1. Set to preheat your oven at 350 degree Fahrenheit or 175 degree Celsius.
2. Take a skillet or pan and heat it over medium flame. Add the margarine to it. Add all the ingredients except lemon juice to it and sauté them. Cook the ingredients until the onions have turned translucent.
3. Now once you have cooked the onions through, add the lemon juice to it.
4. Take a casserole dish and place the ingredients into the dish.
5. Bake the ingredients in the preheated oven for about 30 minutes. You are ready to serve the food hot.

Apple rice salad

Ingredients

- 1 tablespoon olive oil
- 2 tablespoons balsamic vinegar
- 2 teaspoons honey
- 1 tablespoon orange peel (Finely shredded)
- 2 teaspoon brown or Dijon mustard
- ¼ teaspoon garlic powder
- 2 medium apples (Chopped)
- 2 cups cooked rice of any kind (Chilled)
- 1 cup celery (Thinly sliced)
- 2 tablespoons unsalted sunflower seeds (Shelled)

Method

1. Take a small bowl and add the olive oil, vinegar, mustard, honey, garlic powder and orange peel. Stir them well together and keep this bowl aside.
2. Toss until well mixed. Take a larger bowl than the previous one and add the apples, rice, celery and sunflower seeds. Stir them all together until they are well mixed.
3. Pour in the dressing sauce over the salad of rice in the larger bowl and mix and stir them until the rice mixture is well coated with the dressing.
4. Serve the salad immediately after making it or you can cover it and store it in the refrigerator for about 24 hours.

Triple peas salad

Ingredients

- 1 cup sugar snap peas
- 1 cup fresh or thawed frozen sweet peas
- 1 cup snow peas

Vinaigrette:
- 1 teaspoon soy sauce (Reduced sodium)
- 1 teaspoon fresh lime zest
- ¼ cup fresh lime juice
- 2teaspoons fresh ginger (Chopped)
- 1 tablespoon hot sesame oil
- ½ cup Canola oil (Can substitute grape seed oil)
- 1 tablespoon sesame seeds
- Freshly cracked coarse black pepper (According to taste, for garnishing)

Method

1. Add the sesame seeds to a skillet or pan and lightly toast them, stirring them frequently for about 3-5 minutes.
2. Turn the flame to high and take a large pot to make boiling hot water. Blanch the 3 different peas for about 2 minutes. Drain all the hot water, before adding them to a bowl of cold water. Use a strainer to strain all the water from the peas.
3. Take another small bowl and add black pepper, soy sauce, lime zest and juice. Whisk it thoroughly for about 1-2 minutes to have it well blended.
4. Keep whisking the mixture in the bowl before adding ginger to it. Pour in the canola or grape seed oil little by little before adding sesame oil. Mix it all well by whisking it thoroughly.
5. Take a larger bowl and add the pea mixture to it. Pour in the dressing sauce over it, followed by sesame seeds and black pepper to taste. Make sure to mix everything well. You are ready to serve once you garnish it with a little more black pepper.

Broccoli pancakes

Ingredients

- 3 cups broccoli florets
- 2 large eggs
- ½ cup onion
- 2 tablespoons olive oil
- 2 tablespoons all-purpose white flour

Method

1. Take the broccoli and dice it and chop up the onions.
2. Add the diced broccoli to a small amount of water and boil it for about 5 minutes and drain the water completely.
3. Take the eggs and break them in a bowl. Beat them up nicely before adding the flour, mixing it well with the eggs.
4. Now once the flour and eggs have been mixed, add in the broccoli and onion to it and mix it well by stirring continuously.
5. Take a frying pan or skillet and heat some olive oil in it.
6. Take a spoon and pour the broccoli and onion mixture spoon by spoon into the hot olive oil, making about 4 portions or 8 portions, in case you want to make smaller latkes.
7. Take a spatula and flatten the latkes with it and fry them until brown on both of the sides.
8. Drain on a paper towel to soak up extra oil. Using a paper towel, drain and soak up the extra oil in the latkes. You are ready to serve it hot.

Carrot and apple casserole

Ingredients

- 6 large carrots
- 5 tablespoons all-purpose flour
- 4 large apples
- 2 tablespoons brown sugar
- ½ cup apple juice
- 3 tablespoons butter
- ½ teaspoon ground nutmeg

Method

1. Set your oven to preheat at 350 degree Fahrenheit or 175 degree Celsius.
2. Peel up the carrots and apple before slicing them. Take a medium pot and about 1 quart of water to it. Make it boil. Add the carrots to it and make it boil for about 5 minutes or until it becomes tender. Drain the water well from the carrots.
3. Take a large casserole dish and layer the carrots and apples inside it.
4. Take a bowl and add brown sugar, flour and nutmeg to it. Mix it using a fork and add some butter to it and mix that in as well. This will make up for the crumb topping.
5. Take the carrots and apples in a bowl that is microwaveable or a baking sheet and pour and drizzle some of the flour mixture on top of it before adding a little of the juice onto the bowl as well.
6. Put the apple and carrots in the preheated oven for about 50 minutes or until the carrots and apples have become tender and the topping has turned golden brown.

Cranberry cabbage

Ingredients

- 300 g of whole berry cranberry sauce (Canned)
- 1 medium head red cabbage
- ¼ teaspoon ground cloves
- 1 tablespoon fresh lemon juice

Method

1. Take a large pan or skillet and add lemon juice, cranberry sauce and cloves to it. Heat it. Bring this mixture to a simmer.
2. Add the cabbage to the melted cranberry sauce. Mix them well. Bring this mixture to a boil before reducing the flame to make the mixture simmer. You will have to cook until the cabbage has become tender. Keep stirring it frequently. Serve the food hot.

Grape juice dumplings

Ingredients

- 1/2 cup all-purpose white flour
- 3/4 teaspoon baking powder
- 1 teaspoon sugar
- 1/8 teaspoon salt
- 1/2 tablespoon margarine
- 1 and a 1/4 cup grape juice
- 1 cup water

Method

1. In a medium bowl combine flour, baking powder, sugar, salt and shortening. Add 1/2-cup grape juice and mix into stiff dough.
2. Roll dough very thin on a floured board and cut into strips 1/2" wide and 1" long.
3. Mix 1-cup grape juice with 1-cup water in a saucepan and heat to a boil.
4. Drop dough pieces into boiling grape juice and cook for 10 to 12 minutes.
5. Serve dumpling with small amount of liquid.

Sweet and Sour cucumbers

Ingredients

- 3 medium cucumbers
- 1 medium white onion
- 1/4 cup sugar
- 1/2 cup white wine vinegar
- 1/4 teaspoon black pepper
- 1/4 teaspoon salt (optional)

Method

1. Slice cucumbers and onions about 1/8-inch thick. Place in a large bowl.
2. Combine sugar and vinegar. Mix until sugar is dissolved completely. Add additional sugar or vinegar to desired taste.
3. Pour over cucumbers and onion. Add salt and pepper.
4. Cover bowl with plastic wrap and set in refrigerator at least 2 hours.
5. Serve in small salad bowls as a salad or snack.

Veggie pizza

Ingredients

- 1/2 cup red onion
- 1/2 cup green bell pepper
- 1/2 cup mushroom pieces
- 1/2 cup pineapple tidbits
- 1/2 cup part skim shredded mozzarella cheese
- 2 tablespoons grated Parmesan cheese
- 1 cup Roasted Red Pepper Tomato Sauce
- Pizza Dough

Method

1. Dice onion; chop bell pepper.
2. Prepare Easy Pizza Dough and Red Pepper Tomato Sauce recipes.
3. Preheat oven to 425° F.
4. Shape pizza dough to make two flat 12" pizza crusts.
5. Spread 1/2 cup Roasted Red Pepper Tomato Sauce over each pizza.
6. Top with red onion, mushrooms, bell pepper and pineapple.
7. Sprinkle mozzarella and Parmesan cheeses on top.
8. Bake for 12 to 16 minutes until bubbly and browned.

Bread crumbed green beans

Ingredients

- 1-pound frozen French style green beans

- 1 tablespoon oil
- 1/2 cup onion
- 1 garlic clove
- 2 teaspoons dried dill weed
- 1 tablespoon lemon juice
- 1 teaspoon Worcestershire sauce
- 1/3 cup plain bread crumbs
- 2 tablespoons unsalted butter

Method

1. Preheat oven to 400° F.
2. Chop onion and mince garlic.
3. Cook green beans in microwave according to package directions.
4. In a medium skillet, heat oil and sauté onion with garlic, until onion is translucent.
5. Add dill weed, lemon juice and Worcestershire sauce and stir to mix.
6. Add green beans and toss. Place in a casserole dish.
7. Melt butter and mix with bread crumbs. Sprinkle over green bean mixture and bake for 5 to 10 minutes to brown.

Healthy chicken tortillas with vegetables

Ingredients

- 8 flour Tortillas (Six-inch piece each)
- 60g red pepper (Chopped)
- 60g green pepper (Chopped)
- 120g Onion (Chopped)
- 2 tablespoons canola oil
- 80g cilantro (Chopped)
- 350g chicken breasts (Boneless, cut into 1-inch strips)
- 2 Teaspoons chili powder
- ¼ teaspoon black pepper
- 1/2 teaspoons cumin
- Salt to taste (low sodium)
- 2 tablespoons lemon juice
- Foil (for heating tortillas)

Method

1 Set your oven to preheat at 300 degree Fahrenheit or 150 degree Celsius.

2 Using a foil, you can wrap the tortillas in it.

3 Put the foil wrapped tortillas in the preheated oven and heat them for about 10 minutes.

4 Take a non-stick frying pan or skillet and add about 2 tablespoons of canola oil in it. Turn the flame to medium and heat the oil.

5 Now to the heated oil, pour in the chicken, seasoning it with black pepper, cumin, salt, and lemon juice and chilli powder. Turn the heat to high and fry the ingredients in the pan for about 5 minutes.

6 Now, add in the chopped onions and peppers to the other ingredients in the frying pan.

7 Cook the ingredients for 5 more minutes until the chicken has become juicy and has been fully cooked through. Now you can add in chopped cilantro to the frying pan or skillet.

8 Take the tortillas and add the chicken and vegetable mixture to them in perfect portions to fill up the tortillas. Garnish the prepared tortillas with fresh chopped cilantro and enjoy the food.

Smoked mackerel plate

Ingredient

- 200g smoked mackerel fish (Fillet, without skin)
- 1 lemon
- 2 spring onions (Finely sliced)
- 100g cream cheese
- Pepper
- 1 tablespoon creamed horseradish

Method

1. Take the mackerel fish and chop it up to fine pieces.
2. Take a bowl large enough for mixing and add in the cream cheese, chopped mackerel, cream horseradish, spring onions and lemon zest to it. Mix them all together.
3. Now, once everything has been mixed, add in the juice of 1 lemon and mix it up to form a paste that is coarse. Add in the pepper to it according to your taste to season it well.
6. Now your smoked mackerel cheese spread is ready to eat. You can use this as a dip or to make sandwiches with it.

Low potassium lasagna

Ingredients

- 1 tablespoon olive oil
- 1 onion (Diced in small pieces)
- 250 g chicken (Minced)
- carrots (grated)
- 75g all-purpose flour
- 75g butter (Low fat)
- 1 teaspoon English mustard
- cloves of garlic (Crushed)
- 750 ml soya milk
- 400g chopped tomatoes (Canned)
- 100 ml water
- 50 ml vegetable stock
- 250g lasagna sheets
- 15g mozzarella (Grated) (Optional)
- Pepper to taste
- 1 teaspoon oregano

Method

1. Set your oven to preheat at 200 degree Fahrenheit or 95 degree Celsius.

2. Take a large skillet or frying pan and heat some olive oil in it. Heat the oil by turning the flame to medium heat.

3. Now add in the minced chicken to the oil. Add in pepper as well according to your taste.

4. Sauté the chicken in the pan for about 6 minutes. Make sure to turn the chicken brown. Once you have done that, you can take the chicken off the pan and set it aside.

3. Now add in the onions and vegetables to the frying pan and cook for another 10 minutes. Let the heat be medium. Once you see that the vegetables are cooked through and have become soft, you can remove it from the pan and set it aside.

4. Let the heat still be medium and add in the butter to the saucepan. Make sure that the butter doesn't burn. Add the flour and mustard to this butter and stir and mix it to form a paste.

5. Now, when the flour and mustard has been mixed, add in the soya milk. Make sure to add it little by little and to stir it all in while doing so. This should be done at medium heat as well. Once all the soya milk has been added, it will form a white sauce. Take 6-7 minutes to help it simmer and cook it thoroughly. You will have to keep checking it and stirring it at regular intervals so that it doesn't burn.

6. Now take a frying pan and skillet and heat it. Add in garlic and sauté it for about 2 minutes. Add in the vegetables after that along with tomatoes, chicken and stock. Cook the mixture until the liquid has dried up a little.

7. Take a dish for baking and spread up the tomato sauce on the bottom of the dish. The lasagne sheets are to be assembled on top of the tomato sauce. Spread a little more of the tomato sauce on top of this sheet and then add about one-third of the white sauce on top of it.

8. Repeat the previous step until all the lasagne sheets and the sauce has been used up.

9. Finish the assembling of the lasagne with a layer of white sauce.

10. On top of it, add some grated mozzarella, according to your taste and put this dish inside the preheated oven for baking. This will take about 30 minutes.

11. Once you see that the top layer of your lasagne has turned golden, you will know that it is ready to serve.

Spaghetti Bolognese

Ingredients

- 1 tablespoon olive oil
- 1 onion (Finely chopped)
- 200g minced beef
- 4 large mushrooms (Sliced)
- 400g chopped tomatoes (Canned)
- 1 carrot (Grated)
- 230ml of low salt vegetable stock
- ½ teaspoon Worcestershire sauce
- 2 tablespoons tomato puree
- 1 tablespoon freshly ground black pepper
- 300g whole meal spaghetti
- 1 teaspoon dried basil (Optional)

Method

1. Take a large saucepan or skillet and add some olive oil to it. Heat the oil at medium flame. Pour in the minced beef along with the onions. Fry the ingredients for about five minutes, frequently stirring and mixing them. Make sure to have turned the meat brown and the onions have become soft.

2. Pour in the carrots and mushrooms, mixing them in with the beef and cook it for another one minute. Add in the vegetable stock, tinned tomatoes, Worcestershire sauce, tomato puree, basil and freshly ground pepper. Mix them in with the other ingredients and bring the mixture to a boil. Reduce the heat and allow it to simmer once it has boiled. The simmering would continue for 15-20 minutes until you see that the sauce has become thick enough. Keep it aside.

3. Boil some salted water in a deep saucepan. Boil the spaghetti in the salted water according to the instructions on the packaging. Drain the salted water so that the spaghetti is dry enough.

5. You are almost ready to serve. Divide the spaghetti in four dishes or portions of your choice and add the Bolognese sauce that you made on top of the spaghetti in portions of your choice. You are ready to serve.

Chicken and olive casserole

Ingredients

- 1 tablespoon of vegetable or olive oil
- 1 large onion (Sliced)
- 800g chicken breast
- cloves garlic (Minced)
- 375ml low salt chicken stock
- 400g chopped tomatoes (Tin)
- 1 tablespoon dried sage
- ½ teaspoon sugar
- ½ tablespoon dried thyme
- 2 tablespoons balsamic vinegar
- Pepper
- 1 cup of olives in brine (Black or green or a mixture)

Method

1. Take a deep pan and spray it with some oil. Heat the pan on medium flame and add in the chicken. Cook the chicken until it has browned and then remove the chicken from the pan to set it aside.

2. Now, to the pan add in the onions andgarlic. Sauté the ingredients until they have become tender and soft. Pour in the chicken stock, tomatoes, thyme, sage, balsamic vinegar, sugar and olives. Bring this mixture to boil and then lower the heat to simmer the mixture for a couple more minutes.

3. Check the seasoning of the liquid mixture before adding in the chicken to the pan again. Cover the pan and simmer it gently for about 1 hour.
 4. Do not make the casserole boil because it will make the chicken hard. Make sure to simmer it with a gently bubble so as to leave the chicken tender and juicy.
 6. Serve the casserole with boiled rice and a side of vegetables.

Chicken and lemon casserole

Ingredients

- 2 tablespoons honey
- 2kg chicken thighs or drumsticks (Skinless)
- 1 lemon zest
- 1 lemon juice
- 1 lemon (Sliced into thin rounds)
- Salt
- Freshly ground black pepper
- 80g butter
- 4 garlic cloves (Crushed)
- 1 tablespoon vegetable or olive oil
- 500ml hot low salt chicken stock
- 2 tablespoons of dried thyme (optional)

Method

1. Set your oven to preheat at 400 degree Fahrenheit or 200 degree Celsius.

2. Take a bowl and add in the lemon zest, honey and lemon juice. Whisk them all together until everything has been mixed thoroughly. Now, add in the chicken pieces and toss and turn them until they have combined with the honey mixture. Place the bowl aside for 10 minutes for the marinade to enter the pores of the chicken.

3. Use a flame proof casserole and pour in the 40g butter along with half of the olive oil and heat it over medium flame. When the butter foams, add in half of the marinated chicken and fry it over the medium flame for about 5-6 minutes. Keep turning the chicken occasionally until it has turned golden brown. Set this batch aside and pour in rest of the butter and oil along with the marinated chicken. Repeat the same process as before and set this batch aside as well.

4. Once you have set the pieces of chicken aside, add in the lemon slices, garlic cloves and residual juices of the marinade to the pan and scrape the bottom of the pan with the back of the wooden spoon to take off the burnt bits stuck there. Stir the ingredients well so they are mixed. Add in the chicken that you had set aside and also add the hot chicken stock along with the thyme and stir it well to mix it together. Make sure to boil the mixture before putting it inside the preheated oven for about 30-35 minutes or until you see the chicken has become tender and has been cooked perfectly.

5. Once you are done baking it, put the chicken pieces aside on another warm plate and strain the lemon sauce into a saucepan. Use a fine sieve to do it as you press the garlic pulp with a wooden spoon through the sieve. Turn the flame to high and simmer the lemon sauce for about 5-10 minutes or until the liquid has reduced to a consistency of your choice or has become thin syrup.

7. Pour in the lemon sauce over the chicken casserole that you prepared and you are ready to serve.

Pan fried pork chop with creamy leek sauce

Ingredients

- 2 pork chops
- 1 tablespoon of vegetable or olive oil
- Knob unsalted butter
- 1 garlic clove (Peeled and chopped)
- ½ leek (Washed and sliced)
- sprigs of thyme (Leaves only)
- 50ml milk
- 150ml double cream
- 1 tablespoon fresh parsley (Chopped)

Method

1. Heat a griddle or frying pan until hot. Brush the pork chop with oil and add to the pan to cook for six minutes. Turn the chop over and cook for a further six minutes, or until browned and cooked through. When cooked, the juices will run clear when pierced with a sharp knife. Remove from the heat and set aside to rest for three minutes.

2. For the leeks, heat the oil and butter in a pan and sauté the garlic with the leek and thyme leaves for 3-4 minutes, to soften.
3. Stir in the milk, cream and parsley, then reduce the heat and simmer gently for a further 6-8 minutes, stirring occasionally.
4. Spoon the creamed leek sauce over the pork chop and serve.

Chili Con Carne

Ingredents

- 1 tablespoon of vegetable or olive oil
- 1 onion (Diced)
- garlic cloves (Chopped)
- 250g chicken mince
- Pepper
- ½ to1 tsp. chili flakes (To taste)
- 400g tin of chopped tomatoes
- 300ml of low salt beef or vegetable stock
- ½ tsp. dried mixed herbs
- ½ tsp. of smoked paprika (Optional)
- 400g tin red kidney beans (Drained and rinsed)
- 200g long grain rice or basmati rice

Method

1. Heat a large saucepan over a medium heat. Add the oil and, once hot fry the onion for five minutes, or until soft and translucent. Once soft, add the garlic and cook for two minutes.
2. Add the chicken mince, along with a good pinch of pepper. Mix well and cook for 5-6 minutes, or until there are no raw bits of meat. Add the chilli flakes, tomatoes, stock, dried mixed herbs and smoked paprika if using. Stir to mix well and bring to a simmer.
3. Pour in the drained kidney beans and simmer gently for 30 minutes, or until the chilli con carne is thickened and rich. Taste and adjust the seasoning as necessary.
4. Meanwhile, cook the rice according to the packet instructions.
5. Serve the chilli con carne on top of the rice.

Blueberry Spareribs

Ingredients

- 1,5 kg spareribs
- Brown Sugar ¼ cup
- Flour 3 Tbsp.
- Dry Mustard ¼ tsp.
- Ground cloves ¼ tsp.
- Blueberry sauce 355 ml
- Vinegar 2 Tbsp.
- Lemon juice 1 Tbsp.
- Water 2 cups

Method

1. Place ribs on broiler rack. Broil until brown.
2. Turn to brown other side. Pour off drippings and rinse ribs under warm water.
3. Place ribs in casserole dish. Mix sugar, flour, mustard and cloves in saucepan.
4. Add remaining ingredients.
5. Cook and stir over medium heat until slightly thick.
6. Pour sauce over ribs.
7. Cover. Bake 3500F for 1 hour, uncover for last 15-20 minutes.

Grilled Fish in Foil

Ingredients

- 1-pound fish fillets (Fresh or frozen) (If frozen thaw it)
- 2 tablespoons margarine (No salt added)
- Pepper to taste
- 1 medium onion (Thinly sliced)
- 1 lemon (Cut into wedges)

Method

1. Preheat outdoor grill for medium heat On 4 large buttered squares of aluminum foil, place equal amounts of fish.
2. Sprinkle each serving of fish with margarine (season well) and pepper.
3. Top each serving with onion slices and lemon wedge (squeeze lemon wedge over fish fillet first).
4. Tightly wrap fillets in foil (to prevent leaking) and place on grill Grill 5 to 7 minutes on each side or until fish flakes with fork.

Chef's Note: Thick fish fillets may take longer to cook.

Baked Herbs Chicken

Ingredients

- 4 chicken breasts (Fresh)
- 2 tablespoons herbed seasoned flour (Recipe given)
- 2 tablespoons butter
- ½ cup low sodium chicken stock

Method

1. Dredge chicken in seasoned flour
2. Melt butter, cook chicken until browned, approximately 3-5 minutes each side.
3. Pour chicken stock and cook, stirring until lightly thickened.
4. Reduce heat to medium and cook, covered for 3-4 minutes each side or until chicken is no longer pink.

For oven-baked:

1. Place chicken in a shallow dish and sprinkle with seasoned flour.
2. Pour ½ cup water onto chicken and bake at 400ºF, basting occasionally, for approximately 45 minutes or until chicken is no longer pink.

Herbed-Seasoned Flour:

Mix together: ½ cup flour, 1 teaspoon oregano, 2 teaspoons thyme, 2 teaspoon basil1 teaspoon tarragon, 1 teaspoon paprika and ½ teaspoon ground black pepper

Linguine with Garlic and Shrimp

Ingredients

- 2 ½ quarts water
- ¾ pound linguine pasta (Uncooked)
- 2 tablespoons olive oil
- ½ pound shrimps (Peeled and cleaned)
- 1 cup flat-leaf parsley
- 1 Tbsp. lemon juice
- Black pepper to taste

Method

1. Boil water in a large pot.
2. Add pasta and cook for 10 minutes or until tender.
3. While cooking pasta, separate garlic cloves, leaving skin on.
4. Heat cloves in frying pan over medium heat, stirring frequently.
5. Garlic is ready when it darkens and becomes soft to touch. Skin will be easy to remove.
6. Remove garlic from pan and peel off skin.
7. Heat olive oil in the frying pan and return peeled garlic to the pan.
8. Cook garlic until golden. (Cloves can be cut in half or left whole).
9. Add parsley and shrimp and cook 1 to 2 minutes, until shrimp turns pink.
10. Drain pasta and reserve 1 cup of liquid.
11. Add pasta to pan with shrimp and garlic.
12. Mix all ingredients together and add the reserved cup of liquid.
13. Add lemon juice, black pepper, mix and serve.

Onion Smothered Steak

Ingredients

- 1/4 cup flour
- 1/8 teaspoon pepper
- 1 and a ½ lb. round steak, ¾ -inch thick
- 2 tablespoons oil
- 1 cup water
- 1 tablespoon vinegar
- 1 clove garlic (Minced)
- 1 bay leaf
- ¼ teaspoon dried thyme (Crushed)
- 3 medium onions (Sliced)

Method

1. Cut steak into 8 equal servings. Combine flour and pepper and pound into meat.
2. Heat oil in a skillet and brown meat on both sides. Remove from skillet and set aside. Combine water, vinegar, garlic, bay leaf and thyme in the skillet. Bring to a boil.
3. Place meat into this mixture and cover with sliced onions.
4. Cover and simmer 1 hour.

Pork Souvlaki

Ingredients

- Pork 454g (Cut in 1 inch cubes)

- Oil ¼ cup
- Lemon Juice 3 Tbsp.
- Oregano (Ground) 1 tsp.
- Black Pepper 1/4 tsp.
- Garlic clove (Minced) 1 large

Method

1. Trim fat from pork and cut in cubes.
2. Set aside. In a bowl, add remaining ingredients and mix well.
3. Add pork to marinade mixture in bowl and let sit 1-4 hours.
4. Stir fry pork in a pan over medium heat for 7-10 minutes until browned.
5. Or
6. Place pork on skewers and grill over medium heat on barbeque until done turning once during cooking.

Kidney Friendly Meatloaf

Ingredients

- 2 tablespoons onion
- 20 square saltine-type crackers (Unsalted tops)
- 1-pound lean ground beef (10% fat)
- 1 large egg
- 2 tablespoons 1% low-fat milk
- 1/4 teaspoon black pepper
- 1/3 cup catsup
- 1 tablespoon brown sugar
- 1/2 teaspoon apple cider vinegar
- 1 teaspoon water

Method

1. Preheat oven to 350° F.
2. Finely chop onion. Place crackers in a large zip-top bag and crush with a rolling pin.
3. Coat a loaf pan with nonstick cooking spray.
4. In a large bowl, combine crushed crackers, onion, ground beef, egg, milk and black pepper. Mix well.
5. Place mixture into loaf pan. Bake for 40 minutes.
6. To make topping, mix catsup, brown sugar, vinegar and water in a small bowl.
7. Remove cooked meatloaf from oven and cover with sauce.
8. Return pan to oven and bake for 10 minutes or until internal temperature reaches 160° F.
9. Slice into 6 portions and serve.

Renal Diet Beef Meal

Ingredients

- 2 tablespoons vegetable oil
- 1-pound lean ground beef
- 1 cup onion (Chopped)
- 2 cups rice (Cooked)
- 1 and a ½ teaspoons chili con carne seasoning powder
- ⅛ Teaspoon black pepper
- ½ teaspoon sage

Method

1. Heat oil; add beef and onion. Cook, stirring occasionally until browned.
2. Add rice and seasonings. Mix together.
3. Remove from heat.
4. Cover and let stand 10-14 minutes

Parsley Burger

Ingredients

- 1-pound lean ground beef or ground turkey
- 1 tablespoon lemon juice
- 1 tablespoon parsley flakes
- ¼ teaspoon black pepper
- ¼ teaspoon ground thyme
- ¼ teaspoon oregano

Method

1. Mix all ingredients thoroughly.
2. Shape into 4 small patties about ¾" thick.
3. Place on lightly greased skillet or broiler pan.
5. Broil about 3" from the heat for 10-15 minutes, turning once.

Italian Beef Open Sandwich

Ingredients

- 4 chopped steaks (4-ounces each)
- 1 tablespoon lemon juice
- 1 tablespoon Italian seasoning
- 1 tablespoon black pepper
- 1 tablespoon vegetable oil
- 1 medium onion (Sliced into rings)
- hoagie rolls (Sliced)

Method

1. Combine meat with lemon juice, Italian seasoning and black pepper.
2. Heat oil in frying pan over medium heat.
3. Brown seasoned steaks on both sides until tender. Remove and drain on paper towels.
4. Lower heat; add onion and sauté until onions are tender.
6. Serve open-faced on sliced hoagie roll, topped with onion rings.

Grilled Pork Chops

Ingredients

- 2 tablespoons vegetable oil
- ¼ cup all-purpose flour
- 1 teaspoon black pepper
- ½ teaspoon sage
- ½ teaspoon thyme
- 4 four-ounce lean pork chops (fat removed)

Method

1. Preheat oven to 350°F.
2. Grease baking pan with vegetable oil.
3. Mix flour, black pepper, thyme and sage.
4. Dredge pork chops in flour mixture and arrange in baking pan.
5. Place in oven and let brown on both sides about 40 minutes or until tender.
7. Remove from oven. Serve hot.

Lemon Herbs Beef Tacos

Ingredients

- 1-pound skirt or flank steak (Falda)
- 3 limes
- 2 teaspoons lemon pepper herb seasoning blend
- 2 teaspoons garlic powder
- 1/4 cup cilantro
- 1/4 cup onion
- 3 garlic cloves
- 2 tablespoons olive oil
- 8 flour tortillas (6" size)
- 1/2 cup queso fresco Mexican cheese

Method

1. Marinate steak in shallow dish with juice of 2 limes, lemon pepper and garlic powder, from 30 minutes to overnight.
2. Finely chop cilantro; dice onion and garlic. Make salsa by mixing cilantro, onion, garlic and juice of 1 lime. Cover and refrigerate.
3. Heat 2 tablespoons oil over medium high heat. Slice steak thinly and cook until well done, approximately 3 minutes per side.
4. Preheat oven to 350° F.
5. Place equal amounts of cooked steak, about 1-1/2 ounces, in each flour tortilla.
6. Top each taco with one tablespoon crumbled queso fresco.
7. Wrap each taco in aluminum foil and bake 5 to 8 minutes or until tortillas are warm.
8. Remove from oven. Top each taco with salsa and enjoy

Lemon Pepper Grilled Salmon

Ingredients

- 1-pound fresh salmon fillets
- 1 teaspoon salt-free lemon pepper seasoning
- 1/4 cup lemon juice
- Liquid margarine spray

Method

1. Prepare fresh salmon by sprinkling with salt-free lemon pepper seasoning.
2. Squeeze a small amount of lemon juice over the fish.
3. Spray with 3-4 sprites of liquid margarine spray.
4. Place on preheated grill and cook over medium heat for 15 to 20 minutes or until fish reaches desired doneness. Serve hot.

Seafood Delight

Ingredients

- 1 cup crabmeat (Boiled)
- 1 cup shrimp (Boiled)
- 4 tablespoons green pepper (Chopped)
- 2 tablespoons green onions (Chopped)
- 1 cup celery (Chopped)
- ½ cup frozen green peas
- ½ teaspoon black pepper
- ½ cup mayonnaise
- 1 cup bread crumbs

Method

1. Preheat oven to 375ºF.
2. Combine all ingredients except bread crumbs in a bowl.
3. Place in a greased casserole dish.
4. Top with bread crumbs.
5. Bake for 30 minutes.

Steak Patties

Ingredients

- 1-pound chopped steak/lean ground beef/Chicken/Turkey
- 1 small onion (Chopped)
- ½ cup green pepper (Chopped)
- 1 teaspoon black pepper
- 1 egg
- 1 tablespoon vegetable oil
- ½ cup water
- 1 tablespoon corn starch

Method

1. Mix together meat, onion, green pepper, black pepper, and egg. Form into patties.
2. Heat oil in skillet, add patties and cook on both sides.
3. Add half of water and simmer for 15 minutes. Remove patties.
4. To meat drippings, add remaining water and corn starch. Simmer while stirring to thicken gravy.
5. Pour gravy over steak and serve hot.

Soupy Chicken Noodles

Ingredients

- 1 pound chicken parts
- 1 teaspoon red pepper
- ¼ cup lemon juice
- 1 teaspoon caraway seed
- ½ cups water
- 1 teaspoon oregano
- 1 tablespoon poultry seasoning
- 1 teaspoon sugar
- 1 teaspoon garlic powder
- ½ cup celery
- 1 teaspoon onion powder
- ½ cup green pepper
- 2 tablespoons vegetable oil
- 1 cup egg noodles
- 1 teaspoon black pepper

Method

1. Rub chicken parts with lemon juice.
2. In a large pot, combine chicken, water, poultry seasoning, garlic powder, onion powder, vegetable oil, black pepper, red pepper, caraway seed, oregano, and sugar together.
3. Cook 30 minutes or until chicken is tender.
4. Add remaining ingredients and cook for an additional 15 minutes. Serve hot.

Renal Friendly Fish Fingers

Ingredients

- Cooking spray
- 1 cup whole wheat, plain, or Panko dry breadcrumbs
- 1 cup whole grain or plain cereal flakes
- 1 teaspoon lemon pepper
- ½ teaspoon garlic powder
- ½ teaspoon paprika
- ¼ teaspoon salt
- 2 large egg whites (Beaten)
- ½ cup all-purpose flour
- 3 tilapia fillets (1 pound) (Cut into ½ by 3" strips)

Method

1. Preheat oven to 450°F.
2. Set a wire rack on a baking sheet; coat with cooking spray.
3. Place breadcrumbs, cereal flakes, lemon pepper, garlic powder, paprika, and salt in a food processor or blender. Process until finely ground. Transfer to a shallow dish.
5. Place beaten egg whites in a second shallow dish and flour in a third shallow dish.
6. Dredge each strip of fish in the flour, dip it in the egg and then coat all sides with the breadcrumb mixture. Place on the prepared rack. Coat both sides of the breaded fish with cooking spray.
7. Bake until golden brown and crisp, about 10 minutes.

Beef Enchilada

Ingredients

- 1-pound lean ground beef
- 1/2 cup onion, chopped
- 1 teaspoon cumin
- 1/2 teaspoon black pepper
- 1 garlic clove, chopped
- 12 corn tortillas
- 1 can enchilada sauce

Method

1. Preheat oven to 375 degrees.
2. Brown meat in frying pan.
3. Add onion, garlic, cumin and pepper. Continue cooking. Stir until onions are soft.
4. In another pan fry tortillas in a small amount of oil.
5. Dip each tortilla in enchilada sauce.
6. Fill with meat mixture and roll up.
7. Place enchilada in a shallow pan and top with sauce and cheese if desired.
8. Bake until cheese is melted and enchiladas are golden brown.
9. Served with sour cream, sliced olives, or other topping of your choice.

Chef's Note: Use Chicken instead of beef for Chicken enchiladas

Apple Pork Chops With Spiced Sauce

Ingredients

- 1-pound pork chops
- 2 tablespoons butter
- 1/4 cup brown sugar
- 1/4 teaspoon salt
- 1/4 teaspoon pepper
- 1/4 teaspoon nutmeg
- 1/4 teaspoon cinnamon
- 2 medium tart apples

Method

1. Preheat oven to broil.
2. Peel, core, and slice apples.
3. Broil pork chops in the oven, 4 to 5 minutes on each side.
4. While pork chops are cooking, melt butter in skillet and stir in brown sugar, salt, pepper, nutmeg, cinnamon and apples.
5. Cover and cook until apples are tender and sauce begins to thicken.
6. Spoon sauce over cooked chops and serve.

Pork & Beef Baked Meatballs

Ingredients

- 1-pound lean ground pork
- 1-pound lean ground round beef
- 1/2 cup frozen spinach
- 1 large egg
- 1-1/2 teaspoon dried basil
- 1-1/2 teaspoon dried parsley
- 1 teaspoon garlic powder
- 1/2 teaspoon red pepper flakes
- 1/2 cup dried breadcrumbs

Method

1. Preheat oven to 400 F.
2. In a bowl combine ground pork, ground beef, spinach and seasonings. Add 1/4 cup of the bread crumbs and combine.
3. Roll meat mixture into 24 meatballs.
4. Place remaining bread crumbs on a plate and roll meatballs to coat.
5. Place each meatball into an individual miniature muffin cup. Bake for 20 minutes or until cooked.

Beef Pizza

Ingredients

- 1 and a 1/4 teaspoons dry yeast
- 1 and a 1/2 cups warm water
- 2 tablespoons olive oil
- 1 tablespoon sugar
- 2 cups all-purpose flour
- 3 ounces low-sodium tomato paste
- 1/4 teaspoon garlic powder
- 2 tablespoons Italian seasoning
- 1/4 cup onion
- 1/4 cup green bell pepper
- ½ -pound ground beef
- ¼ teaspoon black pepper
- ¼ teaspoon crushed red pepper
- 6 ounces shredded mozzarella cheese

Method

1. Preheat oven to 425° F.
2. Dissolve yeast in 1 cup warm water. Stir in 1 tablespoon olive oil, sugar and flour to make dough. Place in a greased bowl, cover and set aside.
3. Combine tomato paste, 1/2 cup water, garlic powder, Italian seasoning and remaining oil in a small saucepan and simmer for 5 minutes.
4. Chop onion and bell pepper.
5. Brown meat with black pepper and crushed red pepper in a skillet. Drain off fat. Add onion and green pepper.
6. Spray a pizza pan or a 17" x 14" baking sheet with non-stick cooking spray. Press dough onto pan or sheet. Spread sauce, meat mixture and cheese over dough. Bake for 20 minutes or until dough and cheese is golden brown.
7. Cut into 8 slices.

Honey Mustard Turkey

Ingredients

- 3 and a 1/2 pounds turkey breast (With skin and bone-in)
- ¼ cup butter (Melted)
- ¼ cup honey
- 1 tablespoon mustard
- 2 teaspoons curry powder
- 1 teaspoon garlic powder

Method

1. Place turkey breast skin side up on a rack in a shallow roasting pan. Insert meat thermometer in center of thickest part of the turkey breast.
2. Bake at 350° F until thermometer reaches 170° F (about 1-1/2 hours).
3. Combine butter, honey, mustard, curry powder and garlic powder. During the last 30 minutes of cooking, brush turkey with glaze several times.
4. Remove turkey from pan and let stand 15 minutes before slicing.

Haddock with Cucumber Salsa

Ingredients

- 1 small ear fresh corn
- ½ cup cucumber
- ¼ cup red onion
- 1 garlic clove
- ¼ cup red bell pepper
- ¼ teaspoon cayenne pepper
- 3 tablespoons fresh cilantro
- • ½ tablespoons lime juice
- 1-pound fresh haddock
- ½ teaspoon black pepper
- ½ teaspoon garlic powder
- ½ teaspoon onion powder

Method

1. Turn on broiler.
2. Cook cleaned ear of corn in a grill pan or on a hot grill until grill marks are apparent. Stand ear of corn upright. Using a sharp knife, cut kernels from stalk.
3. Peel and dice cucumber. Dice onion, bell pepper; peel and mince garlic; chop cilantro.
4. In a bowl, combine cucumber, onion, garlic clove, red pepper, cayenne pepper, cilantro, grilled corn kernels and 1-1/2 tablespoons lime juice. Place in the refrigerator and allow flavors to blend.
5. Cut fish into four 4-ounce fillets. Score fillets lightly with a sharp knife. Season with pepper, garlic powder and onion powder. Drizzle fillets lightly with remaining 3 tablespoons lime juice. Arrange on baking sheet lined with parchment.
6. Place baking sheets under broiler and cook until golden brown or cooked thoroughly. (Internal temperature of fish should reach 145° F.)

Chicken Tortilla Wrap with Pineapple Salsa

Ingredients

- 8 flour tortillas (6" size)
- 2 tablespoons canola oil
- 360g chicken breast (Skinless and boneless)
- ¼ teaspoon black pepper
- 2 teaspoons chili powder
- 1/2 teaspoons cumin
- 2tablespoons lemon juice
- 1/4 cup chopped green pepper
- 1/4 cup chopped red pepper
- 1/2 cup chopped onion
- 1/2 cup chopped cilantro
- 1/2 cup Pineapple Salsa

Method

1. Preheat oven to 300° F. Wrap tortillas in foil; heat in oven for 10 minutes.
2. Cut chicken breasts into 1" strips.
3. Place oil in nonstick frying pan over medium heat; add chicken, seasonings and lemon juice. Cook for 3 to 5 minutes.
4. Add peppers and onion to frying pan; cook for 3 to 5 minutes more or until chicken is no longer pink and juice run clear. Add cilantro to chicken mixture.
5. Divide chicken mixture between tortillas; fold tortillas over. Serve each with 1 tablespoon of pineapple salsa.

Crisped Catfish

Ingredients

- 1 egg white
- 1/2 cup all-purpose flour
- 1/4 cup cornmeal
- 1/4 cup panko bread crumbs
- 1 teaspoon salt-free Cajun seasoning
- 1-pound catfish fillets

Method

1. Heat oven to 450° F.
2. Spray the surface of a flat, nonstick baking sheet with cooking spray.
3. Beat the egg white in a shallow bowl until very soft peaks form. Do not over-beat.
4. Place flour on a sheet of wax paper.
5. On a separate sheet of wax paper, combine the cornmeal, panko and Cajun seasoning.
6. Cut catfish fillet so you have a total of 4 pieces. Dip the fish in the flour and shake off excess.
7. Dip flour coated fish in the egg white, then roll in the cornmeal mixture.
8. Place fish on the baking pan, and repeat steps 6 to 9 with all the fish fillets.
9. Spray the tops of the fish fillets with cooking spray and bake for 10 to 12 minutes, until the bottom of the fillets are browned and the fish is sizzling. Remove pan from the oven and turn fish over.
10. Return fish to oven and bake about 5 minutes longer until fillets are browned and crisp.

Garlic Cream Shrimp

Ingredients

- 240g bowtie pasta (Uncooked)
- 3 tablespoons unsalted butter
- 3 garlic cloves
- ¼ cup onion (Minced)
- 1-pound raw shrimp
- ½ cup whipped cream cheese
- ¼ cup half & half creamer
- ¼ cup white wine
- 2 tablespoons fresh basil

- $^1/_8$ teaspoon black pepper

Method

1. Shell and devein shrimp.
2. Boil 3 quarts water in a large saucepan. Add 3 cups dry bowtie pasta; cook 12 minutes, then drain.
3. While pasta is boiling, mince garlic and onion. Melt butter in a skillet over medium heat. Add garlic and onion and cook 1 minute. Add shrimp and cook until it turns orange, 1 to 2 minutes (do not overcook).
4. Remove shrimp from skillet and set aside. Reduce heat to low. Add cream cheese to skillet and stir with onion, garlic and butter to make a sauce.
5. Add half & half creamer and stir. Add the wine and stir until smooth. Return cooked shrimp to the sauce and stir to coat.
6. Drain pasta, divide onto 4 plates and top with shrimp and garlic sauce. Season with 1/2 tablespoon chopped fresh basil and black pepper.

Grilled Chicken with Pineapple

Ingredients

- 1 cup dry sherry
- 1 cup pineapple juice
- 1 tablespoon reduced-sodium soy sauce
- 1 and a ¼-pound chicken breast (Bone in and skinless)
- 4 pineapple rings

Method

1 Place all ingredients except pineapple into a zip-lock style bag.
2 Refrigerate and marinate overnight.
3 Place marinated chicken on a barbecue grill or indoor grill and cook for 15 to 20 minutes until done.
4 Discard unused marinade.
5 During the last few minutes, place pineapple on grill top for 2 minutes each side to heat. Serve on top of each chicken breast.

Jerk Chicken

Ingredients

- 6 medium green onions
- 1 small onion
- 2 teaspoons fresh ginger
- 3 garlic cloves
- 2 habanero or 1 scotch bonnet chili pepper
- 2 tablespoons white vinegar
- 1 tablespoon canola oil
- 2 tablespoons brown sugar
- 1 teaspoon kosher or sea salt
- 2 teaspoons fresh thyme
- 1 teaspoon ground allspice
- ¼ teaspoon black pepper
- ¼ teaspoon ground nutmeg

- $1/_8$ teaspoon cinnamon
- 1 and a 1/2 pounds chicken thighs (Skinless and boneless)

Method

1 Coarsely chop the green and yellow onions. Peel and chop the ginger. Mince the garlic cloves. Seed and chop the hot peppers.

2 Place all ingredients, except chicken, in a food processor and process until smooth.

3 Place chicken and blended mixture in a dish or large zip-top bag. Seal and refrigerate to marinate for 3 to 24 hours.

4 Remove chicken from the container and discard remaining marinade.

5 Heat a grill on medium-high heat. Oil the grill rack, then add chicken and cook on each side for about 10 to 12 minutes. Chicken should reach 165° F before removing from the grill.

Red apple pork ribs

Ingredients

- 1 large onion
- 1 medium red apple
- 3 pounds baby back pork ribs
- 1 tablespoon brown sugar
- 1 teaspoon Creole seasoning
- 1 and a ½ tablespoons olive oil
- ½ cup water

- $^1/_3$ cup prepared barbecue sauce

Method

1. Preheat oven to 225° F.
2. Cut onion into 1/2" slices. Core apple and cut into 1/2" slices.
3. Combine brown sugar and Creole seasoning in a small bowl; set aside.
4. Place ribs in a 9" x 13" glass baking dish (cut ribs in half to fit into pan).
5. Rub olive oil onto both sides of ribs, then repeat using brown sugar and Creole seasoning mixture.
6. Place onion and apple slices on top of ribs.
7. Pour 1/2 cup water into dish and cover tightly with foil.
8. Bake for approximately 5 to 6 hours. Remove foil and brush ribs with 1/3 cup barbecue sauce. Bake uncovered for an additional 45 minutes or more at 325° F until temperature of ribs reaches 185 ° F.
9. Remove from oven. Carefully drain liquid, and discard onion and apples.
10. Cut ribs into individual pieces and serve immediately, or cool and freeze for a later date.

Honey and mustard chicken

Ingredients

- $^1/_3$ cup mayonnaise

- 1 and a 1/2 tablespoons deli-style mustard
- 1 tablespoon honey
- 1 teaspoon apple cider vinegar
- 2 green onions (Chopped)
- 1-pound chicken breasts (Skinless and boneless)

Method

1. In a small bowl, combine mayonnaise, mustard, honey, vinegar and green onions to make a sauce. Reserve 1/4 cup to serve with cooked chicken.
2. Grill 1 pound boneless, skinless chicken breasts over medium heat. Brush with honey mustard sauce and turn several times until chicken is cooked through.
3. Remove from grill and serve with reserved honey mustard sauce.

Your choice of grilled or baked trout

Ingredients

- 2 pounds rainbow trout fillets
- 1 tablespoon cooking oil
- 1/2 teaspoon salt
- 1 teaspoon salt-free lemon pepper
- 1/2 teaspoon paprika

Method for baked trout

1. Preheat oven to 350° F.
2. Wash and dry fillets. Rub lightly with oil.
3. On a large sheet pan, place the fillets skin down.
4. Combine seasonings in a small bowl. Sprinkle evenly over fillets.
5. Bake uncovered for 10 to 15 minutes or until the trout fillets flake easily with a fork.

Method for grilled trout

1. Preheat grill on high heat.
2. Spray or brush fillet side of the trout fillets lightly with oil. Combine seasonings in a small bowl. Sprinkle evenly over fillets.
3. Place trout directly on the grill, fillet side down. Cook for 4 minutes. Spray or brush skin lightly with oil. Turn fillets over and cook until fish flakes easily with fork, about 3 to 5 minutes.

Pork cucumber rings

Ingredients

- 2 cucumbers
- 1-pound ground pork
- 1 egg
- 1 teaspoon cornstarch
- 2 teaspoons sugar
- 3 tablespoons red wine
- 1 tablespoon garlic powder
- 1 tablespoon fresh ginger (Minced)
- 1 and a 1/2 tablespoons Mrs. Dash Lemon Pepper seasoning blend
- 1 and a 1/2 tablespoons Mrs. Dash Chicken Grilling Blend
- 1 teaspoon dried basil
- 1 teaspoon dried parsley
- ¼ cup water

Method

1. Peel cucumbers and cut each cucumber horizontally into 4 round pieces. Remove seeds from the middle of each cucumber round to make it hollow in the center.
2. In a mixing bowl combine ground meat with egg, cornstarch, sugar, wine, garlic powder, ginger, Mrs. Dash seasonings, basil and parsley.
3. Add 1/4 cup water gradually into ground meat mixture and mix well until water is absorbed.
4. Stuff the cucumber round with ground meat stuffing. Place each piece in a food steamer and steam about 15 minutes until meat is done.

Chicken tortilla pizza

Ingredients

- 60g cream cheese
- ¼ cup broccoli
- ¼ cup red onion
- ¼ cup fresh mushrooms
- 2flour tortillas (8-inch size)
- I Can't Believe It's Not Butter!® Spray
- 4tablespoons marinara sauce
- 60g grilled chicken

Method

1. Preheat oven to 400° F.
2. Set cream cheese out to soften. Chop broccoli; slice onion and mushrooms.
3. Spray both sides of each flour tortilla with I Can't Believe It's Not Butter!® spray and place on an aluminum foil covered baking tray.
4. Bake both tortillas in the oven until golden brown, flipping tortillas as needed, for approximately 5 to 10 minutes.
5. Remove tortillas from the oven and spread each with 1 ounce of cream cheese.
6. Add 2 tablespoons marinara sauce to each tortilla and spread until covered.
7. Slice chicken and layer 1 ounce of chicken on each tortilla then top with vegetables.
8. Reheat in 400° F oven for approximately 5 minutes or until vegetables are cooked.
9. Remove from oven, cut into quarters and serve.

Vegetable and chicken soup with gnocchi dumplings (renal diet)

Ingredients

- 2 pounds chicken breast
- 1-pound gnocchi (Ready-made)
- 60ml grape seed oil
- 1 tablespoon Chicken Base (Low sodium)
- 5lchicken stock (Low sodium)
- 120g fresh celery (Small diced)
- 120g fresh onions (Small diced)
- 120g fresh carrots (Small diced)
- 60g fresh parsley (Finely chopped)
- 1 teaspoon black pepper (Crushed)
- 1 teaspoon Italian seasoning

Method

1. Add oil to a stockpot over high heat.
2. Fry the chicken in hot oil until it achieves a golden brown colour from all sides.
3. In the stockpot add diced carrot, celery, onion and continue to cook with the chicken until the vegetables become translucent.
4. Then add chicken stock to the chicken and vegetable mixture.
5. Bring it to a boil and cook for 20– 30 minutes over medium-low heat.
6. After 20– 30 minutes reduce the heat and add the chicken base, crushed black pepper and Italian seasoning.
7. Add the gnocchi and stir continuously to mix well.
8. Cook for another 15 minutes.
9. Switch off the flame, garnish with finely chopped parsley and serve hot.

Carrot and Coriander Soup (Renal Diet)

Ingredients

- 1 tablespoon olive oil
- 1 onion (Sliced)
- 450g carrots (Sliced)
- 1 Bundle Fresh coriander leaves (Roughly chopped)
- 2 liters vegetable stock (Low salt)
- 1 bay leaf
- 1 tablespoon coriander powder
- Black pepper (Freshly Ground)
- ½ bundle fresh parsley (Roughly chopped)

Method

1. Take a thick bottom pan and heat oil.
2. Add onion and carrots and sauté for 3 to 4 minutes or until soft.
3. Add coriander powder and sauté for 1 min.
4. Add the vegetable stock and bay leaf and bring to the boil.
5. Cook over a low flame until vegetables are tender.
6. Remove the bay leaf and blend the soup and strain.
7. Bring the soup to a boil and add fresh coriander and parsley.
8. Garnish it with chopped coriander and serve it with crusty bread.

Chicken soup

Ingredients

- 1 tablespoon olive oil
- 1 leek (Roughly chopped)
- 3 medium carrots (Roughly chopped)
- 2 medium potatoes (Peeled, roughly chopped)
- 1 liter chicken stock (Low salt)
- 1 tablespoon cornflower (Optional)
- 300g leftover roast chicken (Shredded)
- 3 tablespoons Greek yogurt.
- 1 tablespoon lemon juice

Method

1. Take a large pot of water and add leeks, carrots and potato.
2. Boil the vegetables until tender.
3. Drain the cooking water and add chicken stock.
4. Blend the soup using a hand blender to desired consistency.
5. Make slurry by adding cold water with corn flour and add it to the soup and simmer until the soup turns to a thicker consistency. (Only follow this step if you want a thick soup)
6. Add the shredded roasted chicken to the soup and simmer for 5 minutes.
7. Top it with Yogurt, lemon juice and fresh coriander leaves(optional) and serve hot with bread croutons.

Beef and Barley Stew

Ingredients

- 1 cup uncooked pearl barley
- • pound lean beef stew meat (Cut into 1and a ½ inch cubes)
- 2 tablespoons flour
- ¼ teaspoon black pepper
- ½ teaspoon salt
- 2 tablespoons oil
- ½ cup diced onion
- 1 large stalk celery (Sliced)
- 1 clove garlic (Minced)
- 2 carrots (Sliced ¼ inch thick)
- 2 bay leaves
- 1 teaspoon onion herb seasoning

Method

1. Soak barley in 2 cups of water for 1 hour.
2. Place flour, black pepper and stew meat in a plastic bag. Shake to dust stew meat with flour.
3. 3. quart pot and brown the stew meat. Remove meat from pot. Sauté onion, celery and garlic in meat drippings for 2 minutes.
4. Add 2 quarts of water and bring to a boil.
5. Return meat to the pot. Add bay leaves and salt. Return heat to a simmer.
6. Drain and rinse barley, then add to the pot.
7. Cover and cook for 1 hour. Stir every 15 minutes.
8. After 1 hour add carrots and onion seasoning.
9. Simmer for another hour. Add additional water if needed to prevent sticking.
10. Portion each serving with 1 and a half cup soup, three pieces of meat , a slice of bread

Beef and Vegetable stew

Ingredients

- 1-pound beef stew
- ½ cups water
- 1 cup raw sliced onions
- ½ cup frozen green peas
- 1 teaspoon black pepper
- ½ cup frozen okra
- ½ teaspoon basil
- ½ cup frozen carrots (Diced)
- ½ teaspoon thyme
- ½ cup frozen corn

Method

1. In a large pot, place beef stew, onions, black pepper, basil, thyme and water.
2. Cook for about 45 minutes.
3. Add all frozen vegetables; simmer on low heat until meat is tender. Serve hot.

Chicken Stew

Ingredients

- 3 tablespoons vegetable oil
- 2 pounds chicken breast (Cut in bite size pieces)
- 1 cup sliced onions
- ¾ cup green peppers
- 2 cloves garlic (Minced)
- 2 tablespoons all-purpose flour
- Two 300 ml cans low-sodium chicken broth
- One 300g bag frozen carrots
- ¼ teaspoon dried basil
- ¼ teaspoon black pepper
- One 1kg bag frozen sliced okra

Method

1. Heat 2 tablespoons of oil in Dutch oven; add chicken and sauté over medium high heat.
2. Remove chicken and set aside. Add remaining 1 tablespoon of oil
4. Add and sauté onion, pepper and garlic.
5. Add flour and cook 2-3 minutes, stirring constantly.
6. Add chicken and broth, cook until boiling.
7. Add carrots, basil and black pepper, cover and simmer for about 10 minutes.
1. Gravy will thicken as it simmers.
8. Add okra and cook for 5-10 more minutes.
9. Serve over hot white rice.

Mixed Vegetable Corn Soup

Ingredients

- 1 cup fresh green beans
- ¾ cup celery
- ½ cup onion
- ½ cup carrots
- ½ cup mushrooms
- ½ cup frozen corn
- 1 medium Roma tomato
- 2 tablespoons olive oil
- ½ cup frozen corn
- 4 cups low-sodium vegetable broth
- 1 teaspoon dried oregano leaves
- 1 teaspoon garlic powder
- ¼ teaspoon salt

Method

1. Remove tips and strings from the green beans and cut into 2-inch pieces. Dice the celery, onion, carrots, mushrooms and tomato.
2. In a large pot heat the olive oil and sauté the celery and onion until tender.
3. Add the remaining ingredients and bring to a boil. Reduce heat to a simmer and cook for 45 to 60 minutes.

Roasted Chicken Soup

Ingredients

- 1 prepared rotisserie chicken
- 8 cups low-sodium chicken broth
- 1/2 cup onion
- 1 cup celery
- 1 cup carrots
- 3 tablespoons fresh parsley

Method

1. Remove chicken from bones and chop into bite-sized pieces. Measure 4 cups for the soup.
2. Pour chicken broth in a large stock pot; bring to a boil.
3. Chop onion; slice celery and carrots.
4. Add chicken and vegetables to stock pot.
5. Bring to a boil and cook approximately 15 minutes until noodles are done.
6. Garnish with chopped parsley.

Kidney Friendly Cabbage Soup

Ingredients

- 1 tablespoon olive oil
- ½ of a sweet onion (Chopped)
- 2 teaspoons garlic (Minced)
- 6 cups water
- 1 cup sodium-free chicken stock
- ½ head green cabbage (Shredded)
- 2 carrots (Diced)
- 2 medium tomatoes (Diced)
- Black pepper, freshly grounded, to taste
- 2 tablespoons fresh thyme (Chopped)

Method

1. In a large saucepan over medium-high heat, heat the olive oil.
2. Add the onion and garlic, and sauté until softened, about 3 minutes.
3. Stir in the water, chicken stock, cabbage, carrots, and tomatoes, and bring to a boil. Reduce the heat to medium-low and simmer until the vegetables are tender, about 30 minutes.
4. Season the soup with black pepper. Serve hot, topped with the thyme.

Apple Cider Vegetable Beef Stew

Ingredients

- 1 and a 1/2 cups potato
- 2 pounds stewing beef cubes
- 7 tablespoons all-purpose white flour
- ¼ teaspoon black pepper
- ¼ teaspoon thyme
- 3 tablespoons canola oil
- 1 and a 1/2 cups carrot
- 1 cup onion
- ½ cup celery
- 1 cup apples (Peeled)
- 2 cups apple cider
- 1 and a 1/2 cups water
- 2 tablespoons apple cider vinegar

Method

1. Dice potatoes into 1/2-inch cubes and soak or double-boil to reduce potassium if you are on a low potassium diet.
2. Mix together 3 tablespoons of the flour, black pepper and thyme.
3. Coat beef with flour mixture.
4. In a skillet heat oil and brown beef pieces. Set aside.
5. Slice carrots, dice onion, celery and peeled apple.
6. In Crock-Pot, layer ingredients as follows: carrots, boiled potatoes, onions, celery, browned beef, and diced apple.
7. Mix together cider, 1 cup water and vinegar.
8. Pour over ingredients in Crock-Pot and cook on low setting for 8-10 hours.
9. Before serving, turn Crock-Pot on high. Mix remaining 4 tablespoons flour with 1/2 cup water. Stir into Crock-Pot to thicken stew.

Long Grain Rice and Chicken Soup

Ingredients

- $^2/_3$ cup long grain and wild rice blend (Uncooked)

- 1 tablespoon onion (Minced)
- 1 tablespoon fresh parsley
- 1 cup carrots
- 250g chicken breast (Cooked)
- 2 tablespoons butter
- ¼ cup all-purpose white flour
- 5 cups low-sodium chicken broth
- 1 tablespoon slivered almonds (optional)

Method

1. Combine rice with 2 cups broth 1/2 cup water. Cook in a rice cooker or on the stove top.
2. Mince onion and parsley. Grate carrots. Chop chicken.
3. Melt butter in a saucepan; add onion and sauté until tender.
4. Blend in flour; gradually add chicken broth.
5. Cook over medium heat, stirring constantly, until mixture thickens slightly.
6. Stir in rice, chicken, and carrots. Simmer 5 minutes.
7. Add almonds and garnish with chopped parsley before serving.

Broccoli Cream Soup

Ingredients

- 2 cups low-sodium vegetable broth
- 3 cups broccoli florets
- 240g silken tofu (Undrained)
- 3 tablespoons corn-starch
- 3 tablespoons nutritional yeast
- 1 teaspoon onion powder
- 1 teaspoon garlic powder
- ¼ teaspoon black pepper

- $1/8$ teaspoon red pepper flakes

Method

1. In a large pot, boil the broccoli florets and tofu (with liquid) in the vegetable broth until tender. Set aside to cool.

2. Carefully pour the cooled contents of the pot into a large mixing bowl and blend until smooth using an immersion blender. Alternately, carefully pour contents of the pot into a large blender. Remove top stopper to allow steam to vent. Blend until smooth.

3. In a small bowl, combine 1-1/2 cups of the soup with the cornstarch. Whisk until smooth.

4. Pour soup back into the pot, add cornstarch mixture and bring to a boil. Stir in nutritional yeast and spices until well combined.

Lamb Stew

Ingredients

- 1 and a ½ pounds boneless lamb shoulder
- ½ teaspoon salt
- ½ teaspoon black pepper
- 1 tablespoon olive oil
- 1 medium onion
- 1/4 cup all-purpose flour
- 3 garlic cloves
- 1 teaspoon dried thyme
- 1/2 cup tomato sauce
- 1 cup stout beer
- 2 cups low-sodium beef broth
- 2 medium carrots
- 2 medium parsnips
- 1 cup frozen peas

Method

1.

1. ½ chunks. Chop the onion and garlic.
 2. Place the lamb pieces on a plate and sprinkle with the salt and pepper. Place flour in a zip top bag. Add lamb and shake to coat meat evenly.
 3. Heat 1 tablespoon of the olive oil over medium heat in a large stockpot or Dutch oven. Add lamb and cook until evenly browned. Remove from the pot and set aside.
 4. Add the onion to the same pot and sauté until translucent. Add chopped garlic and stir for 1 minute. Add 1/2 cup beef broth and stir to deglaze the pot.
 5. Add lamb, beef broth, beer, tomato sauce and thyme to the pot. Bring to a boil, then cover and reduce to low heat. Simmer for 1 hour.
 6. Peel and cut carrots and parsnips into 1-inch pieces. Stir vegetables into stew, cover and simmer for 30 minutes. Add green peas and cook 5 to 10 minutes.

Cool cucumber

Ingredients
- 2 medium cucumbers

- $^1/_3$ cup sweet white onion

- 1 green onion
- ¼ cup fresh mint
- 2 tablespoons fresh dill
- 2 tablespoons lemon juice

- $^2/_3$

cup water
- ½ cup half and half cream

- $^1/_3$ cup sour cream

- ½ teaspoon pepper
- ¼ teaspoon salt (Low sodium)
- Fresh dill sprigs for garnish (Optional)

Method

1. Peel and seed cucumbers. Chop onions and mint. Mince dill.
2. Place all ingredients into a blender and blend until smooth.
3. Cover and refrigerate until chilled.
4. Garnish soup with fresh dill sprigs if desired.

Soup jar

Ingredients
- 3 large reduced-sodium black olives

- $\frac{1}{3}$ cup no salt added, canned chickpeas

- ½ cup frozen or fresh bell pepper and onion strips
- ½ tablespoon Mrs. Dash Garlic & Herb seasoning blend
- ½ teaspoon black pepper
- 1 teaspoon extra virgin olive oil

- $\frac{1}{8}$ teaspoon crushed red pepper flakes (optional)

- 1 tablespoon whole milk ricotta cheese
- ½ cup coleslaw mix

Method

1. Slice the black olives. Rinse the chickpeas.
2. Layer all ingredients in the order listed in a 480g glass jar.
3. Refrigerate until ready to prepare and serve.
4. Remove jar from refrigerator 15 minutes before ready to eat.
5. Pour 150 ml boiling water into the jar, close the lid and shake to combine. Let ingredients set in unopened jar for 2 minutes.
6. Pour contents of jar into a deep, wide bowl. Enjoy!

Ground beef soup

Ingredients

- 1-pound lean ground beef
- ½ cup onion
- 2teaspoons Mrs. Dash lemon pepper seasoning blend
- 1 teaspoon Kitchen Bouquet seasoning and browning sauce
- 1 cup reduced-sodium beef broth
- 2cups water

-

$^1/_3$ cup white rice, uncooked

- 3cups frozen mixed vegetables (corn, green beans, peas and carrots)
- 1 tablespoon sour cream

Method

1. Chop onion. In a large saucepan, brown ground beef with onion. Drain fat.
2. Add seasoning and browning sauce, broth, water, rice and mixed vegetables.
3. Bring to a boil on high heat. Reduce to medium-low heat, cover and cook 30 minutes.
4. Remove from heat, stir in sour cream and serve.

Chili ground beef

Ingredients

- 1 and a 1/4 cups onion
- 3garlic cloves
- 1 and a 1/2 cups hominy
- 1 and a 1/2 pounds lean ground beef
- 1 teaspoon ground cumin
- 1 teaspoon chili powder
- 1 teaspoon Kitchen Bouquet browning and seasoning sauce
- 1 cup reduced-sodium beef stock
- 480g low-sodium canned tomatoes

Method

1. Chop onion and garlic. Drain and rinse hominy.
2. Brown beef in a Dutch oven.
3. Add to beef and sauté until onion is transparent.
4. Add remaining ingredients and simmer for 30 to 45 minutes.
5. Serve with warm bread or crackers.

Pumpkin Pie Crusted Cheesecake for Renal diet

Ingredients

- 1 vanilla wafer pie crust (8-inch piece)
- 1 egg white
- 450g cream cheese
- 60g sugar
- 1 teaspoon vanilla extract
- ½ cup egg substitute
- 120 ml pumpkin (Pureed)
- 1 teaspoon pumpkin pie spice
- 8 tablespoons frozen whipped Topping (Non-dairy)

Method

1. Switch on oven and preheat to 375 F.
2. Take egg white and whisk it until smooth.
3. Apply the egg wash to the Pie crust and bake for 5 minutes.
4. Lower oven temperature to 350F.
5. Take a large bowl and add cream cheese, sugar and vanilla in it.
6. Use a hand blender or mixer at high speed to mix until smooth.
7. Add egg substitute to the mixture.
8. Pour in the pumpkin puree and add pumpkin spice to the mixture.
9. Mix everything until smooth.
10. Take the baked pie crust and pour the pumpkin mixture in it.
11. Bake for 30 to 40 minutes.
12. Take the pie out of the oven and rest it until it cools down.
13. Then refrigerate the pumpkin pie.
14. Cut the pie into desired sized slices.
15. Top each slice with 1 tablespoon whipped topping and serve.

Kidney Friendly Pasty

Ingredients

- 250g of your chosen mince
- 1 medium onion (Finely chopped)
- 1 medium carrot (Peeled and chopped)
- ½ small swede or ¼ large one (Peeled and chopped)
- 2 teaspoons dried parsley
- 120ml low salt stock
- ½ teaspoon of English mustard
- 500g ready-made short crust pastry
- 1 medium egg (Lightly whisked)
- Pepper

Method

1. Preheat the oven to 180°C (160°C Fan)/350°F/ Gas
2. On the hob boil the chopped swede and carrot for 5-10 minutes or until just slightly soft, then drain and discard the water (this helps lower the potassium content of these vegetables). Allow the vegetable to cool.
3. In a separate bowl add the parsley, stock, onion, minced beef and English Mustard.
4. Use a knife to cut the minced beef into small strands and mix the lot together with your hands so that the ingredients are roughly spread evenly throughout the mixture. Season with pepper.
5. Add the cooled down vegetables and gently combine with your mince mixture.
6. Take the pastry and roll it out with a rolling pin to about 3mm thick. Press a saucer over the rolled pastry and cut round it to leave a circle of pastry. You may need to do three circles then reform and re-roll the pastry. Place some of the filling on each circle.
7. Brush a small amount of the egg around the edges of the pastry. Bring two edges of the pastry together to make a 'parcel' and crimp the edges together all the way round.
8. Brush the sides of the pasties with the egg (to give a browned colour during cooking).
9. Put the pasties in the pre-heated oven on a greased baking tray for 55 minutes.

Christmas Cake

Ingredients

- 200g glace cherries (Halved)
- 200g mixed peel
- 100g tinned peaches (Drained and roughly chopped)
- 100g tinned pineapple (Drained and roughly chopped)
- 2eggs (Beaten)
- 1 tablespoon brandy
- 250g plain flour
- 150g self-rising flour
- 200g unsalted butter
- 150g caster sugar
- 1 tablespoon nutmeg
- 2 tablespoons mixed spice

Method

1. Preheat the oven to 150°C/300°F/Gas
2. Grease and line a 7in baking tin.
3. Cream butter and sugar until light and fluffy. Sieve the flour and spices together. Add the eggs and flour alternately to the creamed mixture, mixing well after each addition. Stir in the fruit, peel and brandy. Turn into the tin and cook for 3hours.
4. Ice when cool with white icing but avoid marzipan which is high in phosphate.

Gingerbread Yule Log

Ingredients

- 50g butter (Plus extra for greasing)
- 50g treacle
- 50g golden syrup
- 2 balls of stem ginger (Finely grated)
- 2 tablespoons of the syrup of the grated ginger
- 4 large eggs
- 100g dark muscovite sugar (Plus extra for dusting)
- 100g plain flour
- ½ tsp. baking powder
- 2 tablespoons ground ginger
- ½ tsp. ground cinnamon

For the icing
- 200g butter (Softened)
- 250g icing sugar
- 2tsp. vanilla extract
- 3tbsp. ginger syrup from the stem ginger jar

Method

1. Heat oven to 190C. Grease and line a 20 x 30cm Swiss roll tin with baking parchment, then grease the parchment a little too. Put the treacle, syrup, butter and stem ginger in a pan, heat until melted and stir to combine, then set aside to cool a little.

2. Put the eggs and sugar in a bowl and whisk using an electric hand whisk until light, mousselike and doubled in size– this will take about 10 minutes. Sift over the flour, baking powder and spices, and then pour the melted butter mixture around the sides of the bowel so that it trickles down into the whisked eggs. Very gently fold everything together with a large metal spoon. When just combined pour the mixture into the Swiss roll tin and ease it into the corners. Bake for 12 minutes until just cooked.

3. While the sponge is cooking, lay a sheet of baking parchment big enough to fit the cake on your work surface and dust with a little sugar. Once cooked, tip the cake directly onto the parchment. Use a small serrated knife to score a line about 2cm from one of the shorter ends, making sure you don't cut all the way through – this will help to get a tight roll. Gently roll up from this end, rolling the parchment between the layers. Leave to cool like this on a wire rack to help set the shape.

4. To make the icing, put the ingredients in a bowl and whisk until smooth. Transfer to a piping bag fitted with a large round nozzle or use a plastic sandwich bag and snip off one corner to make a hole about 1cm wide. Unroll the sponge and drizzle the surface with 2 tbsp. ginger syrup. Pipe a layer of ginger buttercream over the inside of the roll, then use the paper underneath to help tightly re-roll into a roulade. Slice off both ends for a neat finish. The buche can be frozen. Defrost at room temperature before continuing.

5. Place the Buche on a serving plate or board. Use the remaining icing to pipe a thick layer over the top of the sponge, zigzagging backwards and forwards to create a tight concertina pattern. Decorate with white pearl sprinkles, if you like. The Buche will keep in a sealed container for up to 5 days, or can be frozen for up to two months.

Syrup Sponge Pudding

Ingredients

- 100g softened unsalted butter
- 100g caster sugar
- 2eggs
- 100g self-rising flour
- 6 tablespoons golden syrup

Method

1. Cream the butter and sugar together in a bowl or food processor.
2. Add one egg and mix carefully with a spoon of flour to prevent curdling. Add the other egg and mix well.
3. Fold in the flour.
4. Measure the syrup into a buttered pudding dish. Spoon the cake mixture on top of the syrup.
6. Cover with buttered foil with a fold to allow for expansion.
7. Bake at 200°C (180°C Fan)/400°F/Gas 6 for 35-40 minutes until a skewer comes out clean.

Blackberry Lemon Muffins

Ingredients

- 1 cup All-purpose flour
- ¾ cup Whole Wheat flour
- ½ cup granulated sugar
- 2 tablespoons Baking powder
- ½ tablespoon Baking soda
- 1 tablespoon Grated lemon or orange peel
- 1 and a ½ cups Coffee Rich
- ½ cup Margarine (Melted)
- 2 egg whites
- 1 cup Fresh or frozen unsweetened blackberries

Method

1. Preheat oven to 375 F.
2. In a large bowl, stir flours with sugar, baking powder, baking soda, and lemon peel until well mixed.
3. In a medium bowl, whisk Coffee Rich® with margarine and egg whites until blended. Stir Coffee Rich® mixture into flour mixture just until combined.
4. Fold in blackberries.
5. Spoon batter into lightly greased, non-stick or paper lined muffin tins.
6. Bake for 20-22 minutes, until lightly golden on top and a toothpick inserted in centre comes out clean.

Quick Canned Pear Dessert

Ingredients

- $^1/_3$ cup unsifted flour

- ¼ cup Sugar
- ¼ cup unsalted Butter or Margarine
- 3 cups canned pears
- 2 tablespoons Lemon juice
- ¼ cup Sherry
- ¼ tsp. Nutmeg

Method
1. Preheat oven to 350 0F

2. In a medium bowl, stir flour and sugar together.
3. With two knives or pastry blender, cut margarine or butter and flour until mixture is crumbly.
4. Set aside. Drain canned pears.
5. Place sliced pears into a well-greased 9-inch pie plate.
6. Sprinkle fruit with lemon juice, sherry and nutmeg; Scatter flour mixture over top.
7. Bake in hot oven for 15 minutes or until browned

Renal Friendly Bran Muffins

Ingredients

- ¼ cup oil
- 1 egg
- 1 tsp. vanilla
- 1/3 cup honey
- 1 cup applesauce or crushed pineapple (Drained)
- 1 cup white flour
- 1 cup wheat bran
- 1 and a ½ tsp. baking soda
- ¼ tsp. cream of tartar

Method

1. Preheat oven to 400ºF and lightly grease muffin tins
2. Mix together, spoon into muffin tins and bake immediately.
3. Cream of tartar and baking soda will only rise once so do not delay getting the muffins into the oven.
4. Bake for 15-20 minutes.
5. Makes 12 muffins

Finland's Stripped Cake

Ingredients

- 3 cups unsifted all-purpose flour
- 1 cup sugar
- 1 teaspoon baking powder
- 1 cup (½ pound) butter or margarine (Softened)
- 2 whole eggs plus 1 egg white
- ½ teaspoon vanilla
- 1 cup jelly or jam (Plum, blackberry, or raspberry jelly, or apricot jam)
- 2 tablespoons sugar

Method

1. Heat oven to 375°F.
2. In a large bowl, combine flour, sugar, and baking powder.
3. Blend in butter with finger tips or pastry blender until mixture resembles cornmeal.
4. Add eggs, egg white and vanilla; work into stiff dough.
5. Divide dough into two balls, one twice the size of the other. On a heavily floured board (¼ to ½ cup flour), roll out the larger ball to 1/8" thickness.
6. Place rolled dough in a cookie pan (11" x 15 ½"), smoothing out to edges and patching corners. Spread jelly over the top.
7. Roll out remaining dough to 1/8" thickness and cut into ½ " wide strips; place strips diagonally across the jelly, ½" apart. Sprinkle sugar over the top. Place in oven.
8. When edges start to brown (about 20 minutes), take pan from the oven, cut off and remove about a 3" strip all around the edges. Return pan to oven, remove after 10 minutes.
9. Cut into 1" x 2" rectangles. Makes 7 dozen cookies.

Lemon Pastry Squares

Ingredients

For crust layer

- ¼ cup powdered sugar
- ⅛ Teaspoon salt
- 1 cup all-purpose flour
- ½ cup unsalted butter

For filling layer

- 1 cup granulated sugar
- ½ teaspoon baking powder
- ⅛ Teaspoon salt
- 2 eggs (Slightly beaten)
- 2 tablespoons fresh lemon juice
- Zest from one lemon

For icing layer

- 2 tablespoons fresh lemon juice
- ¾ cup powdered sugar
- 1 tablespoon unsalted butter (Softened)

Method
For crust layer

1. Mix all ingredients together.
2. Press into ungreased 8" square pan
3. Bake at 350° F for 15 minutes.
4. Remove from oven and spread with the filling layer.
For filling layer

1. Mix all filling ingredients together.
2. Spread evenly on top of baked crust layer.
3. Return to oven, and bake an additional 20 minutes at 350°F.
5. Remove from oven and cool.
For icing layer

1. Mix all ingredients together.
2. When baked crust and filling are completely cool, spread icing over the top.

Classic Lemon Pound Cake

Ingredients

- 2 cups butter or margarine
- 4 cups powdered sugar
- 2 tablespoons grated lemon rind
- 1 teaspoon lemon extract
- 6 eggs
- 3 ½ cups all-purpose flour (Sifted)

Method

1. Preheat oven to 350°F.
2. Using an electric mixer on medium speed, cream butter for 3 minutes, or until light and fluffy.
3. Gradually add sugar and rind; cream thoroughly.
4. Add lemon extract and eggs, one at a time, mixing well after each addition.
5. Gradually add flour; mix well.
6. Pour into greased and floured 10" tube pan or Bundt pan.
7. Bake one hour and 20 minutes or until wooden pick inserted in center of cake comes out clean.
8. Remove from pan and cool.

Glazed Pineapple Cake

Ingredients

For cake

- 3cups sugar
- 1and a ½ cups butter
- 6whole eggs and 4 egg whites
- 1teaspoon vanilla extract
- 3cups all-purpose flour (Sifted)
- One 300g can crushed pineapple (drain and reserve juice)

For glaze

- 1 cup sugar
- 1 stick margarine (½ cup)
- Juice from pineapple

Method

1. Preheat oven to 350°F.
2. Beat together sugar and butter until smooth and creamy.
3. Add eggs and egg whites two at a time, mixing after each addition.
4. Add vanilla.
5. Add sifted flour and mix well.
6. Add drained, crushed pineapple.
7. Bake for 45 minutes to 1 hour.
8. In a medium saucepan, mix together ingredients for glaze. Stir frequently. Bring to a boil, until desired thickness is reached. Pour over top of cake while hot.

Cinnamon Pound Cake

Ingredients

- 3 sticks butter or margarine
- ¼ teaspoons nutmeg powder
- 1 teaspoon Cinnamon powder
- 1 teaspoon vanilla extract
- 1-pound sifted powdered sugar
- 6eggs
- 3 cups all-purpose flour
- Powdered sugar (Garnish)

Method

1. Preheat oven to 325°F.
2. Cream butter in a large bowl until softened.
3. Blend in nutmeg or mace and vanilla extract.
4. Gradually stir in powdered sugar.
5. Add eggs, one at a time, beating well after each addition.
6. Gradually stir in flour.
7. Grease only the bottom and lightly flour a 10" x 4" round tube pan. Do not grease the sides!
8. Bake for 1 hour and 20 minutes or until a cake tester inserted in the centre comes out clean.
9. Allow cake to cool. Sprinkle with powdered sugar when cold.

Barbecue Sauce

Ingredients

- ¼ cup dark corn syrup
- ¼ cup red wine vinegar
- ¼ cup onion (Chopped)
- 1 cup water
- 2 teaspoons dry mustard
- 2 tablespoons tomato paste
- 1 teaspoon Tabasco pepper sauce
- 2 tablespoons vegetable oil
- 1 tablespoon all-purpose flour
- 1 teaspoon Mrs. Dash (of your choice)

Method

1. Mix all ingredients together except vegetable oil and flour in a sauce pan.
2. Mix vegetable oil and flour together in separate container to make paste.
3. Add to sauce pan, cook on low heat until desired thickness is reached.
2. Pour or brush on baked or grilled meats.

Alfredo Sauce

Ingredients

- 1/4 cup olive oil
- 3 tablespoons all-purpose flour
- 1 clove garlic (Minced)
- 2cups rice milk
- 4ounces cream cheese
- 1/3 cup shredded Parmesan cheese
- 1/4 teaspoon ground nutmeg
- 1 tablespoon lemon juice

Method

1. Heat olive oil in a large skillet over medium heat. Add flour and whisk to make a paste then add minced garlic.
2. Slowly add rice milk, whisking constantly to prevent lumps. Let mixture come to a boil and thicken.
3. Add cream cheese and mix well. Remove from heat.
4. Add 1/3 cup Parmesan cheese, nutmeg, and lemon juice. Mix well.
5. Serve over pasta, chicken, steamed vegetables, etc.

Cherry and Apple Spread

Ingredients

- 1 medium tart apple
- 1 cup dried tart cherries
- 1 small red onion (Thinly sliced)
- 1 cup apple cider vinegar
- 1 and a 1/2 cups sugar

Method

1. Quarter and core the apple and cut into thin slices, leaving the skin on.
2. Put the apples and cherries in a heavy saucepan with the onions, vinegar, and sugar. Cook, stirring until the sugar is dissolved and the mixture is beginning to boil.
3. Cover and reduce heat to low and cook until the onions are tender and the dried cherries are plump and tender, about 8-10 minutes.
4. Uncover and bring the heat up to high and boil until the syrup around the fruit is reduced to a shiny glaze, about 5 minutes more. Chutney may be served at once or kept, covered and refrigerated for several days.

Fresh Basil Oil

Ingredients

- 1 and a 1/2 cups fresh basil leaves
- 1 cup olive oil or vegetable oil

Method

1. Rinse and drain 1 1/2 cups lightly packed fresh basil leaves.
2. Pat leaves dry with towel.
3. In a blender or food processor, combine basil leaves and 1 cup olive oil or vegetable oil. Whirl just until leaves are finely chopped (do not puree).
4. Pour mixture into a 1 to 1 1/2 quart pan over medium heat. Stir occasionally until oil bubbles around pan sides and reaches 165 degrees on a thermometer, 3-4 minutes. Be sure the oil is heated to this temperature to kill any bacteria in the mixture.
5. Remove from heat and let stand until cool, about an hour.
6. Line fine wire strainer with two layers of cheesecloth and set over a small bowl.
7. Pour oil mixture into strainer.
8. After oil passes through, gently press basil to remaining oil.
9. Discard basil.
10. Serve oil or store in an airtight container in the refrigerator up to 3 months. The olive oil may solidify slightly when chilled, but will quickly liquefy when it comes back to room temperature.

Salt-Free Barbecue Seasoning Rub

Ingredients

- 1 tablespoon brown sugar
- 1 teaspoon smoked paprika
- 1 teaspoon chili powder
- 1 teaspoon garlic (Granulated)
- 1 teaspoon onion powder
- 1 teaspoon cumin
- ¼ teaspoon dry mustard powder

- $^1/_8$ teaspoon allspice
- $^1/_8$ teaspoon ground red pepper (Optional)

Method

1. In a bowl, blend all ingredients together thoroughly.
2. Rub on pork or chicken before cooking.

Basil Peach Dressing

Ingredients

- 1 fresh peach
- 1 tablespoon fresh shallot
- 3 tablespoons champagne vinegar
- 2 tablespoons extra virgin olive oil
- 2 tablespoons lemon juice
- ½ tablespoon dried basil

Method

1. Peel the peach and remove the pit. Dice the shallot.
2. Place all dressing ingredients into a small blender or food processor. Blend until smooth.
3. Store dressing in an airtight container in the refrigerator for up to 1 week.

Blackberry Sauce for Waffles

Ingredients

- 5 cups fresh blackberries
- ¾ cup sugar
- 1 tablespoon cornstarch
- 1 tablespoon lemon juice

Method

1 Crush berries then combine with 1 cup water and sugar in a large saucepan. Bring mixture to a boil.

2 Combine cornstarch with 2 tablespoons water. Mix well and stir into blackberry mixture. Cook 1 minute over medium high heat to thicken sauce, stirring constantly.

3 Remove from heat and add lemon juice. Chill in refrigerator until ready to serve.

Roasted red pepper tomato sauce (For veggie pizza)

Ingredients

- ½ cup roasted red peppers
- 1 garlic clove
- ½ cup low-sodium tomato sauce
- 2 tablespoons olive oil
- 1 teaspoon dried Italian seasoning
- ¼ teaspoon red pepper chili flakes

Method

1. Drain red peppers and measure 1/2 cup, (approximately 2 whole peppers).

2. Place peppers and garlic in food processor or blender and process until smooth.
3. Add tomato sauce, olive oil and Italian seasonings. Process until well blended. Ready to use on pizza, pasta or as a replacement for tomato sauce in recipes.
4. May be refrigerated 2 to 3 days or frozen until ready to use.

Raspberry Vinaigrette

Ingredients

- ¼ cup fresh lime juice
- 2 tablespoons raspberry vinegar
- 2 tablespoons fresh raspberries
- 2 tablespoons raspberry preserves
- ½ teaspoon fresh tarragon
- 2 teaspoons sugar
- ¼ teaspoon kosher salt
- ¼ cup canola oil

Method

1. Crush raspberries and chop tarragon.
2. Whisk together first 7 ingredients.
3. Slowly whisk in oil until well blended. Serve.
4. Store remaining dressing in a tightly sealed jar and refrigerator until ready to serve. Keeps for up to one week.

Honey chive dressing

Ingredients

- 2 tablespoons fresh chives (Chopped)
- 1 teaspoon fresh ginger root (Grated)
- 2 and a ½ tablespoons fresh lemon juice
- 1 tablespoon honey
- 1 tablespoon reduced-sodium soy sauce
- ½ teaspoon dark sesame oil

Method

1. Chop chives and grate ginger root.
2. In a small bowl whisk all ingredients together.
3. Serve dressing over salad greens or arugula.

Fruit Pizza

Ingredients

- 1 roll of frozen sugar cookie dough
- 250g package cream cheese (Softened)
- 120g Cool Whip nondairy topping
- 1 cup sugar or Splenda equivalent
- Pears (Sliced in half)
- 1 cup pineapple juice
- 2 tablespoons lemon juice
- 2 tablespoons cornstarch
- Nonstick cooking spray
- 1 apple (Cored and sliced thinly) (Put in lemon juice to prevent browning)
- 20 grapes (Both red and green) (Sliced in half)
- medium strawberries (Sliced)

Method

1. Preheat oven to 325°F.
2. Cook sugar, pineapple juice, lemon juice and cornstarch over medium heat until thickened.
3. Slice cookie dough in 1/4" slices. Place close together on pizza pan sprayed with nonstick cooking spray.
4. Bake until brown.
5. Beat cream cheese with cool whip until fluffy. Spread on cooled cookie crust.
6. Arrange fruit slices on top of cream cheese.
7. Pour cooled pineapple glaze over the fruit and put in the fridge for several hours before serving.

Pizza Muffin

Ingredients

- 1 split English muffin
- ¼ cup pizza sauce
- 2 tablespoons shredded mozzarella cheese

Method

1. Toast English muffins.
2. Spread pizza sauce evenly on muffin halves.
3. Sprinkle cheese and add toppings.
4. Place the muffin halves on tray and put into toaster oven, set on broil.
5. Broil for about 5 minutes, watching carefully to remove when cheese is golden and melted.

Baked Stuffed Apple

Ingredients

- 4 apples for baking
- 1 cup apple juice
- ¼ cup brown sugar, packed
- 2 tablespoons Craisins
- Red cinnamon candies

Method

1. Preheat oven to 375ºF.
2. Wash and core the apples. Set aside.
3. Using a square baking pan (9 "x 9" x 1 ¾"), blend the apple juice and brown sugar.
4. Place apples in pan.
5. Fill apple centers with craisins and cinnamon candies.
6. Place pan in the oven. Spoon juice over apples occasionally during baking, to glaze the apples and keep them from drying out.
8. Bake 40 to 45 minutes, or until apples are tender when pierced with a fork.

Kidney Friendly Fried Chicken

Ingredients

- 2 and a ½ pound fryer (Cut as desired)
- 1 tablespoon lemon juice
- 1 cup all-purpose flour
- 1 teaspoon black pepper
- 1 cup corn flakes (Crushed)
- ¼ teaspoon poultry seasoning
- 4 tablespoons vegetable oil

Method

1. Preheat oven to 400°F.
2. Wash chicken parts thoroughly and pat dry; rub with lemon juice.
3. In a small bag, combine flour, black pepper, corn flakes, and poultry seasoning. Shake well.
4. In a shallow baking pan (about 1" deep), grease with vegetable oil.
5. Place chicken in bag of ingredients, using the largest pieces first. Shake well.
6. Arrange coated chicken in pan.
7. Brown in oven 20-30 minutes on each side.

Home Baked Simple Biscuits

Ingredients

- 2 cups all-purpose flour (Sifted)
- 3 teaspoons double acting baking powder
- 2 teaspoons sugar
- ⅓ Cup vegetable shortening
- ¼ cup 1% milk
- ½ cup water

Method

1. Preheat oven at 350°F. Sift dry ingredients into a bowl.
2. Cut in shortening until coarse crumbs form. Make a well in the mixture.
3. Pour milk and water into the well.
4. Stir quickly with a fork until dough follows fork around the bowl.
5. Dough should be soft. Turn dough onto lightly floured surface.
6. 6. 12 times. Roll or pat dough until ½" thick.
7. Dip a 2 ½" biscuit cutter into flour; then cut out 10 biscuits.
8. Bake biscuits on ungreased baking sheet for 12-15 minutes.

Mango Pudding

Ingredients

- 2 Cups Fresh Ripe Mangoes
- 3 Slightly beaten eggs or ¾ cup egg substitute
- ½ Cup 1% milk
- ½ Cup water
- ⅓ Cup onion (Finely chopped)
- 1 Tablespoon butter (Melted)
- 1 Teaspoon granulated sugar
- 1 Teaspoon white or black pepper

Method

1. Preheat oven to 350°F.
2. Combine all ingredients.
3. Pour into a greased 1 ½-quart casserole dish.
4. Place in a shallow pan filled with 1 inch of hot water.
5. Bake 40-45 minutes, or until knife inserted in centre comes out clean.
6. Let stand for 10 minutes at room temperature before serving.

Orange Cookies

Ingredients

- 1 cup unsalted butter or margarine
- 1 cup granulated sugar
- 1 egg
- 1 ½ teaspoons Orange extract
- 1 ½ cup all-purpose flour, sifted

Method

1. Preheat oven to 375°F.
2. Cream butter with sugar.
3. Add egg and lemon extract, beat until light and fluffy.
4. Add flour, mix until smooth.
5. Drop batter by level tablespoon onto ungreased cookie sheet, at least 2" apart.
6. Bake for 10 minutes until brown around the edges.
7. Remove from cookie sheet after the cookies have cooled for a minute.

Diamond Cookies

Ingredients

- 5 cups all-purpose flour
- 2 cups butter
- 1 cup plus 2 tablespoons sugar
- 2 eggs
- 1 teaspoon almond extract
- 2 teaspoons vanilla extract

Method

1. Preheat oven to 400°F.
2. Combine flour, butter and sugar.
3. Add eggs and extracts; mix with a spoon or hand mixer on low speed.
4. Drop cookies onto ungreased baking sheet or use cookie gun.
5. Bake for 5-8 minutes.
6. Cool and serve.

Carrot and Pineapple Cake

Ingredients

For cake

- 1 cup granulated sugar
- ½ cup vegetable oil
- 2 eggs
- 1 ½ cup carrots (Grated or shredded)
- 1 teaspoon vanilla extract
- 2 cups all-purpose flour
- 2 teaspoon baking soda
- 1 teaspoon baking powder
- 2 teaspoons ground cinnamon
- ¼ teaspoon nutmeg
- ¼ teaspoon ground cloves
- 1 cup canned pineapples (Crushed and drained)

For icing

- One 120g bar cream cheese (Softened)
- ¼ cup unsalted margarine (Softened)
- 1 tablespoon vanilla
- 2 cups powdered sugar (Sifted)

Method
For cake

1. Preheat oven to 375°F.
2. Combine sugar, oil and egg; beat well.
3. Add carrots, and vanilla. Beat until smooth.
4. Add remaining ingredients to mixture; mix well.
5. Pour into greased and floured 9" x 13" cake pan.
7. Bake for 30 minutes. Cool in pan 10 minutes. Remove from pan.
8. Garnish with whipped cream or top with icing (optional).
For icing

1. Mix together cream cheese and unsalted margarine. Add vanilla and powdered sugar. 2. Spread over cooled cake. (May need extra powdered sugar to stiffen the icing).

Pineapple Cream Cheese Torte

Ingredients

- ½ cup unsalted butter (Softened)
- ¾ cup sugar (Divided in 1/4 cups)
- 1 cup flour
- 250g cream cheese (Softened)
- 1 egg
- 1 teaspoon vanilla
- ½ of a medium Pineapple (Thinly sliced)
- ½ teaspoon cinnamon

Method

1. Preheat oven to 450 degrees.
2. In a medium bowl, cream butter and 1/4 cup of sugar.
3. Blend in flour.
4. Press into a spring form pan.
5. Beat cream cheese, 1/4 cup of sugar, egg, and vanilla until smooth.
6. Spread into the spring form pan.
7. Toss apples with remaining 1/4 cup of sugar and cinnamon.
8. Arrange apples over cheese filling.
9. Bake for 10 minutes.
10. Reduce oven temperature to 400 degrees and bake for an additional 25-30 minutes until filling is firm and the apples have softened.

Baked Asian Pear Dessert

Ingredients

- ¾ cup nuts (Chopped)
- 1/2 cup unbleached all-purpose flour
- 1/4 cup light brown sugar
- 4 tablespoons granulated sugar (Divided)
- ¼ teaspoon ground cinnamon
- teaspoon ground nutmeg
- 5 tablespoons unsalted butter
- 1 tablespoon corn-starch
- Juice from one lemon
- 3 pounds Asian pears (Peeled & cored)

Method

1. Preheat oven to 375 degrees.
2. Mix nuts, flour, brown sugar, 2 tablespoons granulated sugar, cinnamon, and nutmeg in food processor.
3. Pour melted butter over mixture and mix until mixture resembles wet sand.
4. Whisk remaining 2 tablespoons granulated sugar, cornstarch, and lemon juice in a large bowl.
5. Peel pears, then halve and core. Cut into wedges and then cut in half.
6. Toss pears with sugar mixture and transfer to 8-inch square baking dish.
7. Sprinkle topping over pears.
8. Bake until fruit is bubbling around edges and topping is deep golden brown, about 45 minutes.
9. Cool on wire rack about 15 minutes. Serve.

Blueberry Cream Pie

Ingredients

- 2 cups graham cracker crumbs
- 1 teaspoon cinnamon
- ½ cup unsalted butter (Melted)
- 8 ounces cream cheese (Softened)
- ¼ cup granulated sugar
- 1 teaspoon vanilla extract
- 2 teaspoons lemon juice
- 250g tub of non-dairy whipped cream
- 3 cups blueberries

Method

1 Preheat oven to 375 degrees.
2 In a medium bowl, combine the graham cracker crumbs, cinnamon, and melted butter.
3 Press the mixture evenly into the bottom of a 9 inch round or square baking dish to form a crust.
4 Bake crust for 7 minutes and let cool.
5 In a large bowl, use an electric mixer to mix softened cream cheese with sugar until smooth.
6 Mix in vanilla extract and lemon juice.
7 Gently fold in the whipped topping then fold in the blueberries.
8 Spread mixture evenly over the crust.
9 Cover and chill in the refrigerator for at least 1 hour.

Apple Muffins

Ingredients

- 12 muffin papers
- 1 and a 1/2 cups raw apple
- 2 eggs
- 1 cup sugar
- ½ cup canola oil
- ¼ cup water
- 1 tablespoon vanilla
- 1 and a 1/2 cups all-purpose white flour
- 1 teaspoon baking soda
- 1 and a 1/2 teaspoons cinnamon

Method

1 Preheat oven to 400° F and place muffin papers in muffin pan. peel and cut apple into small pieces.

2 Beat eggs in a large bowl. Add sugar, oil and water; mix well. Add vanilla.

3 In a separate bowl, combine flour, baking soda and 1 teaspoon cinnamon.

4 Stir flour mixture into egg mixture. Batter will be lumpy. Fold in apple pieces.

5 Fill muffin cups 3/4 full. Mix remaining 1/2 teaspoon cinnamon with 1 teaspoon sugar. Sprinkle on top of muffins.

6 Bake for 20 minutes or until lightly browned.

Apple-Pine-Apple Farfel

Ingredients

- 1 cup hot water
- 1 cup Matzo farfel
- ¼ cup sugar
- 2 large apples
- 2 teaspoons ground cinnamon
- 3 egg whites
- ½ cup pineapple chunks

Method

1 Preheat oven to 375° F.
2 Peel, core and shred apples.
3 Spray an 8" x 8" baking dish with nonstick cooking spray.
4 In a large bowl, combine the hot water and farfel.
5 Add the sugar, apples and cinnamon.
6 Beat egg whites to a stiff peak. Fold in the egg whites.
7 Add drained pineapple chunks and stir.
8 Pour mixture into the prepared baking dish and dust the top with more cinnamon.
9 Bake for 45 minutes.

Baked pineapple

Ingredients

- 600g canned crushed pineapple with juice
- 2 large eggs
- 2 cups sugar
- 3 tablespoons tapioca

-
$1/8$ teaspoon salt

- 3 tablespoons unsalted butter
- ½ teaspoon cinnamon

Method

1 Preheat oven to 350°F.
2 Empty crushed pineapple with juice into a bowl.
3 Beat 2 eggs well and add to crushed pineapple.
4 Add sugar, tapioca, and salt to pineapple egg mixture.
5 Pour mixture into 8" x 8" baking dish.
6 Slice butter and place on top of pineapple mixture. Sprinkle cinnamon on top.
7 Bake for 30 minutes. Serve hot or chilled.

Berries Napoleon

Ingredients

- 12 wonton wrappers
- 2 tablespoons granulated sugar
- 1 cup Reddi-Wip fat-free whipped topping
- 1/2 cup raspberries
- 1/2 cup blueberries
- 1 tablespoon powdered sugar

Method

1 Preheat oven to 400° F.

2 Spray the cooking spray on a baking sheet that will fit 12 wonton wrappers.

3 Spread out the wonton wrappers, and spray them with cooking spray.

4 Sprinkle the granulated sugar on wonton wrappers.

5 Bake the wontons for 5 minutes or until golden brown; remove from the baking sheet.

6 Place 6 wonton wrappers on a serving tray.

7 Top each wrapper with 2 tablespoons of whipped topping, 1 tablespoon of raspberries and 1 tablespoon of blueberries.

8 Top the berries with a second wonton wrapper.

9 Sprinkle the tops with powdered sugar. Garnish them with a dollop of whipped topping, fruit and a mint leaf, if desired. Serve immediately.

Blueberry cones

Ingredients

- 120g cream cheese
- 1 and a 1/2 cup whipped topping
- 1 and a 1/4 cup blueberries (Fresh or frozen)
- 1/4 cup blueberry jam or preserves
- 6 small ice cream cones

Method

1 Soften cream cheese. Place in a bowl and beat with a mixer on high until smooth and fluffy.

2 Fold fruit and jam or preserves and whipped topping into the cream cheese.

3 Fill cones, and chill in the freezer until ready to serve.

Three colored pie

Ingredients

- 250g whipped low-fat cream cheese
- ½ cup low-sugar red raspberry preserves
- 3cups Reddi-Wip dairy whipped topping
- 1 prepared graham cracker crust (9" size)
- 1 cup fresh blueberries
- 1 and a 1/2 cups fresh raspberries

Method

1. To make filling, beat whipped cream cheese and preserves until smooth with an electric mixer on medium speed.
2. Fold whipped topping into cream cheese mixture.
3. Spread filling evenly over the bottom of the graham cracker crust.
4. Chill at least 30 minutes in the refrigerator or freezer.
5. Before serving arrange blueberries around outer ring of pie. Layer raspberries around inner ring of pie.
6. Finish decorating with a dollop of whipped topping in the center and a raspberry or strawberry on top.

Apple and caramel salad

Ingredients

- 3 cups Granny Smith apples
- 240g canned crushed pineapple (Packed in juice)
- 240g whipped topping
- ½ cup butterscotch dessert topping

- $1/3$ cup unsalted peanuts
- ¼ cup butterscotch baking chips

Method

1. Wash and core apples, but do not peel. Cut apples into approximately 1" cubes. Thaw whipped topping.
2. Mix crushed pineapple (including juice) with diced apples.
3. In a separate large bowl, combine thawed non-dairy topping with butterscotch flavored dessert topping until evenly distributed.
4. Stir apple/pineapple mixture into the non-dairy topping mixture.
5. Add butterscotch chips and unsalted peanuts to mixture.
6. Stir and serve.

Frozen frooti

Ingredients

- $\frac{1}{3}$ cup maraschino cherries

- 240g canned crushed pineapple
- 240g reduced-fat sour cream
- 1 tablespoon lemon juice
- 1 cup sliced strawberries
- ½ cup sugar

- $\frac{1}{8}$ teaspoon salt
- 3 cups Reddi-Wip dairy whipped topping

Method

1. Chop cherries and drain pineapple.
2. Place all ingredients except whipped topping into a medium-sized bowl and combine until well blended. Fold in whipped topping.
3. Place mixture into a plastic freezable container and freeze 2 to 3 hours until hardened.

Ice cream sandwiches

Ingredients

- 30 graham cracker squares
- 450g canned crushed pineapple in juice
- 8 packets Splenda No Calorie Sweetener
- 1 and a 1/2 cups Procel protein powder
- 1 cup Reddi-Wip dairy whipped topping
- 1 packet Knox unflavored gelatin

Method

1. Line a 13″ x 9-1/2″ baking pan with plastic wrap allowing at least 10″ to hang on both sides of pan.
2. Arrange 15 graham cracker squares in the pan and set aside.
3. Drain pineapple and reserve 1/2 cup of pineapple juice.
4. In alarge mixing bowl, mix crushed pineapple, Splenda® and Procel®, until there are no lumps.
5. Fold in whipped topping then set aside. (The folding motion keeps whipped topping airy and light.)
6. In a small saucepan, boil 1/2-cup pineapple juice. Add 1 packet ofunflavored Knox® gelatin. Mix until dissolved then remove from heat.
7. Lightly fold in gelatin mixture with the whipped topping mixture.
8. Pour mixture evenly over the graham crackers.
9. Top mixture with remaining 15 graham cracker squares.
10. Put plastic wrap from the sides of the pan over the graham crackers. Cover with aluminum foil and seal well. Freeze overnight or at least 6 hours.
11. 11.1/2″ x 2-1/2″ pieces and serve.

Hot Sauce for Steaks

Ingredients

- ¼ cup vegetable oil
- 2 tablespoons all-purpose flour
- 1 teaspoon onion powder
- 2 teaspoons vinegar
- 2 teaspoons sugar
- 1 teaspoon Tabasco sauce
- 2-3 cups water

Method

1. Combine oil and flour in saucepan; stir while cooking until golden brown. Remove from heat.
2. Add onion powder, vinegar, sugar, Tabasco sauce, and water.
3. Return to heat, and continue stirring until thickened.

Chicken Giblet with Seasoning

Ingredients

- 2 cups chicken parts and giblets
- 4 cups water
- 1 cup chopped onion
- ½ cup chopped celery
- ½ cup chopped green peppers
- 1 teaspoon black pepper
- 1 teaspoon poultry seasoning
- 1 teaspoon onion powder
- 1 teaspoon sage

Method

1. Wash chicken parts and giblets and add to water in a large pot.
2. Add onion, celery, green pepper and black pepper.
4. Boil for 30 minutes until tender
5. When done, reserve 2 cups of broth for dressing (remaining broth may be used for giblet gravy on the following page). Let meat cool.
6. Remove meat from bone and add to remaining dressing ingredients.
7. Mix all ingredients together with 2 cups broth from chicken until mixture is moist.
8. Spread into baking pan.
9. Bake at 425°F until golden brown.

Sodium Free Sweet Brown Mustard

Ingredients

- 2 teaspoons corn-starch
- 1 cup cider vinegar
- ½ cup dry mustard
- ½ cup light brown sugar
- ½ teaspoon white pepper (or black pepper)

Method

1. Dissolve corn-starch in small amount of vinegar.
2. Heat remaining vinegar; add mustard, sugar, and pepper. Stir until dissolved.
3. When hot, add corn-starch and cook until thick. Remove from heat.
4. Cover the mixture and let stand at room temperature for 24 hours to develop flavors.

Relish for Burgers

Ingredients

- 2lemons, peeled and quartered
- 1 large onion
- ½ medium green pepper
- 2cups sliced celery
- ¼ cup parsley (Optional)
- ½ cup sugar
- ¼ teaspoon ground mustard
- ⅛ teaspoon allspice
- 1 teaspoon celery seed

Method
1. Chop first five ingredients. Stir in sugar and spices.
2. Cover and place in refrigerator for several hours or overnight to blend flavors.

Chicken Nugget (Renal Diet)

Ingredients

- 2egg whites
- 1 tablespoon water
- 2½ cups ready-to-eat crispy rice cereal
- 1 ½ teaspoons paprika
- ¼ teaspoon seasoning salt
- ⅛ teaspoon garlic powder
- ⅛ teaspoon onion powder
- 1-pound chicken breasts (Skinless and boneless)
- 1 tablespoon butter or margarine (Melted)
- 1 tablespoon reduced-fat ranch dressing (for dipping)

Method

1. In a shallow dish combine egg whites and water.
2. On a large sheet of wax paper combine crispy rice cereal, paprika, seasoning salt, garlic powder and onion powder.
3. Cut chicken into 1 ½" pieces.
4. Dip chicken into egg white mixture, coating all sides. Roll in cereal mixture.
5. Place in a single layer on ungreased baking sheet. Drizzle with melted butter.
6. Bake at 450°F for about 12 minutes or until no longer pink in center.
7. Serve warm with dipping sauce (reduced-fat ranch dressing).

Peppermint Candy Cookies

Ingredients

- ½ cup unsalted butter
- 18 peppermint candies
- ¾ cup sugar
- 1 large egg
- 1/4 teaspoon peppermint extract
- • ½ cups all-purpose flour
- 1 teaspoon baking powder
- ¼ teaspoon salt

Method

1. Set the butter out to soften.
2. Place 12 of the peppermint candies in a zip-top bag and pound with a heavy pan until finely crushed.
3. In a mixing bowl, combine the sugar, butter, egg and peppermint extract. Beat ingredients at medium speed until creamy, scraping the bowl several times.
4. Stir together the flour, baking powder and salt. Turn mixer to low speed and add flour mixture. Beat until well mixed. Hand-stir the crushed peppermint candy into the dough. Refrigerate dough for 1 hour to chill.
5. Preheat the oven to 350° F. Crush the remaining 6 peppermint candies. Line baking sheets with parchment paper.
6. Shape the chilled dough into 3/4-inch balls and place on the baking sheet 2-inches apart. Using your thumb, make an indentation on each cookie and top with about 1/2 teaspoon of the crushed candy.
7. Bake for 10 to 12 minutes or until edges are lightly browned. Remove parchment paper from baking sheet and cool cookies completely. Store in a sealed container with parchment paper or waxed paper between layers of cookies.

Shrimp Stuffed With Crab

Ingredients

- 200g crab meat
- ¼ cup dry breadcrumbs
- 3 tablespoons unsalted butter
- 1 teaspoon celery
- 1 teaspoon parsley
- 1 teaspoon onion and
- 1 teaspoon green bell pepper
- ¼ teaspoon lemon juice
- 3drops hot sauce
- ⅛ teaspoon garlic powder
- ⅛ teaspoon black pepper
- 12 jumbo shrimp (Raw, shelled with tails on)

Method

1. Preheat oven to 450° F.
2. Finely chop crab meat, celery, parsley, onion, and bell pepper.
3. In a bowl mix crab, bread crumbs, 3 tablespoons melted butter, celery, parsley, onion and bell pepper; set aside.
4. Spray a baking sheet with non-stick cooking spray.
5. Wash, devein shrimp and pat dry.
6. Use a sharp knife to cut a 1/2" deep pocket in inner curved side of shrimp from tail along center, leaving 1/2" at end. Do not cut through back of shrimp. Use finger to widen pocket.
7. Use about 2-1/2 tablespoons crab mixture per shrimp. Place portion in hand and squeeze to mold. Place crab in shrimp pocket and distribute to fill. Place shrimp on baking sheet. Repeat, preparing all shrimp.
8. Brush shrimp with melted butter. Bake for 10-12 minutes. Do not overcook.
9. Serve with a side dish of melted unsalted butter if desired.

Cream Cheeseburger

- 1-pound ground beef
- 2 large eggs
- 6 tablespoons cream cheese
- 1 teaspoon dried basil
- 1 teaspoon onion powder
- 1 teaspoon garlic powder
- 4 hamburger buns
- 4 lettuce leaves
- 2 slices onion

Method

1. Mix ground beef, eggs, basil, onion powder and garlic powder together.
2. Separate meat into eight 2-ounce patties.
3. Take 1-1/2 tablespoons of the cream cheese and place on top of a patty.
4. Take another patty and place it on top, to sandwich the cream cheese between the two patties.
5. Repeat this procedure with the remaining patties.
6. Cook in a frying pan or on a grill to desired doneness.
7. Serve burgers on a bun with lettuce, onion and condiment of choice.

Eggplant French Fries

Ingredients

- 1 medium eggplant
- 1 cup 1% low fat milk
- 2 large eggs
- ¾ cup corn-starch
- ¾ cup dry unseasoned breadcrumbs
- 3 teaspoons dry Hidden Valley Original Ranch Salad Dressing and Seasoning Mix
- 1 teaspoon Tabasco hot sauce (optional)
- ½ cup canola oil

Method

1. Peel and slice eggplant into 3/4" sticks, 4" long. Rinse and pat dry.
2. In a medium bowl, mix milk and eggs until well blended; stir in hot sauce.
3. In a wide, shallow bowl, combine cornstarch, bread crumbs, and dry Ranch salad dressing mix.
4. Heat oil in frying pan on high heat.
5. Dip eggplant sticks into egg mixture and then roll each piece in bread crumb mixture.
6. Place in oil, flipping regularly and fry 3 minutes or until golden brown.
7. Drain on paper towels and serve immediately.

Renal Diet Pizza for Kids

- 60g cream cheese
- ¼ cup broccoli
- ¼ cup red onion
- ¼ cup fresh mushrooms
- 2 flour tortillas (8-inch size)
- I Can't Believe It's Not Butter! Spray
- 4 tablespoons marinara sauce
- 60g grilled chicken

Method

1. Preheat oven to 400° F.
2. Set cream cheese out to soften. Chop broccoli; slice onion and mushrooms.
3. Spray both sides of each flour tortilla with I Can't Believe It's Not Butter!® spray and place on an aluminum foil covered baking tray.
4. Bake both tortillas in the oven until golden brown, flipping tortillas as needed, for approximately 5 to 10 minutes.
5. Remove tortillas from the oven and spread each with 1 ounce of cream cheese.
6. Add 2 tablespoons marinara sauce to each tortilla and spread until covered.
7. Slice chicken and layer 1 ounce of chicken on each tortilla then top with vegetables.
8. Reheat in 400° F oven for approximately 5 minutes or until vegetables are cooked.
9. Remove from oven, cut into quarters and serve.

Brewery burger

Ingredients

- 3 tablespoons rice milk
- 5 salt-free soda crackers
- 1 large egg
- 1 teaspoon salt-free herb seasoning blend
- 1-pound ground beef, 85% lean

Method

1. Crush the soda crackers, then combine them with the milk in a bowl. Let stand until crackers are soft.
2. Beat the egg and stir into cracker mixture. Add the herb blend; mix well, breaking up the crackers if necessary. Add the ground beef and mix well.
3. Pat the ground beef mixture into 4 equal-size patties.
4. Grill over medium heat until cooked until the internal temperature is at least 160° F.
5. Serve on a bun with desired toppings, or serve patty with a vegetable and starch of choice.

Creamy turkey burger

Ingredients

- ¼ medium onion

- 2 tablespoons chives
- 1-pound ground turkey 7% fat
- 1 large egg
- 1 tablespoon Worcestershire sauce
- 1 teaspoon minced garlic
- ¼ teaspoon black pepper
- 4 tablespoons sour cream
- 4 cracked wheat hamburger buns

Method

1. Dice the onion and chives.
2. Combine the onion, turkey, egg, Worcestershire sauce, garlic and pepper. Mix well and refrigerate for 1 hour.
3. Form turkey mixture into 4 patties and refrigerate until ready to cook.
4. Grill the turkey patties over medium heat, until well cooked, about 5 to 6 minutes per side. Burgers are done when a meat thermometer registers 165° F.
5. Place each burger on the bottom part of the bun, top with 1 tablespoon sour cream and 1/2 tablespoon chives. Place the other half of bun on top and serve.

Cauliflower Spinach Scrambled Eggs

Ingredient

- 4 whole eggs
- 1 medium cauliflower (frozen)
- 3 bundle fresh spinach
- 1 garlic clove (minced)
- 60g bell pepper, (chopped)
- 60g onion (chopped)
- ¼ teaspoon black pepper (crushed)
- 1 tablespoon coconut oil
- Fresh parsley (finely chopped) for garnishing
- Spring Onion (finely chopped) for garnishing

Method

1. Take the eggs in a bowl and beat them until they have taken a foamy texture and are light and fluffy. Rest it in the bowl for five minutes.
2. Add black pepper to the bowl and mix it nicely.
3. Turn your burner to medium and heat coconut oil in a large skillet or frying pan over it. Heat until the oil has become hot.
4. Add in the onions and bell peppers that have been chopped to the hot oil in the frying pan.
5. Sauté and mix it together until the peppers has taken on a translucent colour and is golden.
6. Add the garlic into the mixture and mix it in quickly so as not to not burn it.
7. Add the cauliflower and spinach to the mixture that has been made in the pan. Sauté the vegetables all together for two minutes over medium flame.
8. Cover the pan with a lid and cook the mixture for another five minutes.
9. Add in the eggs to the veggies and mix it well.
10. When the eggs have been cooked nicely, turn off the flame and pour it into another bowl.
11. You have the option of garnishing it with parsley, spring onions and feta cheese. Serve it hot.

Maple Pancake

Ingredients
- 130g all-purpose flour
- 1 tablespoon regular sugar
- 2 teaspoons baking powder
- 1g salt
- 2 large egg (white part)
- 240ml milk (low-fat)
- 2 tablespoons canola oil
- 1 tablespoon maple extract

Method
1. Take flour, sugar, baking powder and salt in a bowl and mix it together. Set aside the bowl.
2. Take a large mixing bowl and mix egg whites, milk, oil and maple extract. Take egg whites, milk, oil and maple extract and mix them all together.
3. Take the dry mixture and make a cavity in the middle. Pour the egg mixture in it and whisk until the batter is formed.
4. Make the batter a little lumpy.
5. Pour 1/4th cup pancake batter into a hot skillet lightly brushed with canola oil.
6. Cook for 2 min on each side over medium flame or until it is cooked.
7. Flip when there is a slight crust on the edge.
8. Do not press the pancake.
9. Drizzle with honey and maple syrup and serve hot.

Aromatic Apple Porridge

Ingredients
- 35g porridge oats
- 100ml skimmed milk
- 100ml water
- ½ grated apple
- Cinnamon powder (pinch)
- Green Cardamom powder (pinch)

Method
1. Mix water and skimmed milk and heat for 5 minutes over medium heat.
2. Add grated apple and oats. Boil for 5 minutes over medium heat stirring continuously.
3. Sprinkle a pinch of cinnamon powder and cardamom powder and turn of the heat.
4. Garnish with small dices of apple and serve warm.

County Farm's Grilled Cheese

Ingredient
- 25g butter
- 150ml soya milk (unsweetened)
- 175g soft goat's cheese
- 25g flour
- ½ tsp. mustard
- Pepper (according to taste)
- 2 eggs (yolks)
- Bread (4 slices)

Method

1. Take a saucepan and add butter, soy milk and cheese. Gently heat over a low flame and stir until a smooth consistency.
2. Add flour to the butter mixture and bring it to a boil. Stir and bring it to a thick consistency.
3. Add mustard and pepper to the mixture and turn off the flame. Let it rest for 5 minutes.
4. Add two egg yolks and mix well.
5. Take the bread slices and toast it on a griller on one side and spread the cheese mixture on the other side.
6. Then place it on a griller and grill until the cheese melt.
7. Garnish with grated cheese (optional) and serve hot.

Bannock

Ingredients
- 1 and a ½ cup of All-purpose flour
- 2 Teaspoon powdered milk
- 2 Tbsp vegetable oil
- ½ cup water

Method
1. At 400 degree Fahrenheit or 200 degree Celsius, preheat your oven. Take flour, baking powder and powdered milk in a bowl and pour oil as it mix it in. the mixture should look crumbly when done.

2. Water should be added to this crumbly mixture and keep stirring it until it the mixture has been blended evenly.
3. Pour this mixture from your bowl into a pan and bake it for 15 minutes in your oven and serve it hot.

Low Phosphorus Pancakes

Ingredients
- ½ cup Rice Dream or Coffeerich milk substitute
- ½ cup flour
- 1 egg
- 1 tsp. sugar or Splenda
- 1 Tbsp vegetable oil

Method
1. Take a bowl and mix all the ingredients together. Make sure to mix them well.
2. Take margarine according to your needs and melt it at the bottom of your hot pan placed on the flame.
3. Take about 1/4ᵗʰ of the pancake mix and pour it into the pan. Gently tip the mix using the handle of the pan so that it gets evenly spread in the pan.
4. Let it cook for a minute until you see the sides of the pancakes turn golden and then use a spatula to turn it on the other side and let that side cook.
5. Repeat the same steps for all the pancakes that you make.

Potassium Friendly Mashed Potatoes

Ingredients
- Large cooking pot or pan of water
- 2 cups baking potatoes (2 large potatoes)
- ¼ cup polyunsaturated margarine
- ¼ cup Coffee Rich or Original Rice Dream

Method

1. Take the potatoes and peel and slice them into small pieces and add them to a large pot of water.
2. Boil water and add the potatoes to it. Boil them for 10 minutes and then throw out the water.
3. Add cold water to the potatoes and boil it again until it is done. Throw out the used water when it is done.
4. Use a potato masher to mash the potatoes until it has become soft.
5. Add the margarine to the mashed potatoes slowly and also coffee rich or original rice dream, according to your choice. Add them until the mashed potatoes have become creamy.

Low Potassium Hash Brown

Ingredients
- 2 cups potassium friendly mashed potatoes
- 1 egg, beaten
- 1 onion, minced
- 1/8th tsp. pepper
- 2-3 Tbsp Olive Oil

Method
1. Add mashed potatoes, beaten egg and onion to a medium bowl and mix them all together.

Add pepper, according to taste, to the mixture and make sure to have them all mixed nicely.
2. Take olive oil in a frying pan and heat it over medium flame.
3. Take about 1/4th of the mixture in the frying pan and pat it with a spatula to make about a 4 inch circle out of it. They will be about ½ inch thick.
4. Cook the patty until the bottom is browned nicely and has become crisp. It would take about 3-4 minutes. Carefully turn the patty to the other side and brown and crisp it like the other side. Cook it for about the same time.

Vegetable Omelet

Ingredients
- ¼ cups of sliced green pepper
- ½ cup sliced onion
- 1/3 cup frozen mixed vegetables,
- Steamed 2 eggs or 1 egg and 2 egg whites
- 1 Tbsp unsalted margarine
- 2 Tbsp water

Method

1. Take onions and green pepper in a skillet. Sauté them in unsalted margarine. Keep it aside.
2. Take eggs and water in a bowl and beat them. Add this mixture to the skillet with onions and pepper and cook it until it is done nicely.
3. Now when the egg mixture is done, add cooked mixed vegetables to it.
4. Fold the eggs around the vegetables and plate it.

Strawberry Omelette

Ingredients
- 2 cups frozen unsweetened strawberries, thawed
- 1 tablespoon sugar (optional)
- 4 eggs, separated
- 1 tablespoon lemon juice
- 1 tablespoon unsalted margarine

Method

1. Preheat your oven at 375 degree Fahrenheit or 190 degree Celsius.
2. Take thawed strawberries in a bowl and sprinkle them with sugar and let it rest aside.
3. Take another bowl and take egg whites in it. Beat them until it has become stiff.
4. Take another bowl and have the egg yolks in them along with lemon juice. You will have to nicely beat them together as well. Now take the stiff egg whites and add the beaten egg yolks to it. Fold them together until there is no yellow colour of the egg yolks to be seen.
5. Take margarine in a 10 inch or so skillet which is oven proof. Pour the egg white and yolk mixture into this skillet and tilt it from side to side to have it coat all the sides evenly. Cook this at a low flame for 5 minutes.
6. When the mixture has become set at the bottom of your skillet, put it inside the preheated oven. Cook the mixture for another 5 minutes.
7. After the omelette is done, take it out on a hot late and add the sugar sprinkled strawberries to it. Cut the omelette into pie wedges and serve the food hot.

Red Blossom smoothie

Ingredients
- 1 cup cranberry juice cocktail
- 1 cup fresh whole strawberries, washed and hulled
- 2 tablespoons fresh limejuice
- ¼ cup sugar
- 8-9 ice cubes
- Strawberries for garnishing

Method

1. Take strawberries, cranberry juice, sugar and lime juice in your blender and mix them all together.
2. Now add the ice cubes and blend the mixture again until it has become smooth.
3. Pour this mixture into chilled glasses and top it off with strawberries.

Apple crepes

Ingredients
- ½ cup sugar
- 2 whole eggs
- 4 egg yolks
- ¼ cup oil
- 1 cup flour
- ½ cup brown sugar
- ½ teaspoon cinnamon
- 2 cups milk
- 4 apples
- 1/2 teaspoon nutmeg
- 1 stick or 1/2 cup unsalted butter

Method

1 Take whole eggs, flour, egg yolks, sugar, milk and oil in a bowl and mix them all together. Make sure that the mixture does not have any lumps.

2 Take a non-stick skillet or frying pan and heat it over medium flame. Spray the pan with cooking spray.

3 Take the batter in a cup or use a ladle to scoop it onto the pan. Make sure to fill 1/4 th cup of batter. Spread it onto the pan in a swirling technique so that it becomes thin at the bottom of the pan.

4 For 20 seconds, you will have to cook it, before flipping the crepe and cooking that side for another 10 seconds. You can use a rubber spatula for this and you will have to set the crepes aside as you make the filling for the crepes.

5 Take your apples and take out the core of your apples. You will have to slice each of the apples into 12 pieces.

6 Add butter to the pan when it is hot and melt it and further add brown sugar to the pan.

7 Add apples to the pan along with nutmeg and cinnamon. Mix them up in the pan. Cook the apples until they have become tender. Don't make it mushy. When it is done, set them aside to cool down.

8 When your apple mixture is done, take about 2 tablespoons of your mixture and add them to the middle of your crepes. Repeat for each crepe. Roll your crepes into the shape of logs. You are ready to serve.

Mixed berry smoothie

Ingredients
- 2/3 cup silken firm tofu
- ¼ cup of cranberry juice cocktail
- 1/2 cup blueberries, frozen, unsweetened
- 1/2 cup raspberries, frozen, unsweetened
- 1 teaspoon vanilla extract
- 1/2 teaspoon powdered lemonade, such as Country Time

Method

1. Take your cranberry juice and pour it in your blender. Along with it, add in the other ingredients.
2. Blend the ingredients until it has become smooth.
3. You are ready to serve.

Burrito wraps

Ingredients
- ½ of a red bell pepper (Diced)
- 1 and a ½ teaspoons of canola or o live oil
- 8 eggs (Beaten)
- 4 green scallions or onions (Thinly sliced)
- 4 corn tortillas (6-inch)

Method
1. Take a frying pan and heat some oil in it at medium flame.
2. Add green onions or scallions and bell pepper to the oil and cook it until it has become soft. It will take about 3 minutes.
3. Add the beaten eggs to the vegetables and scramble them until the eggs are done perfectly or for about 5 minutes.
4. Take two damp paper towels and the n place your tortillas in between them. You can now place them on a microwaveable plate. Microwave the tortillas for about 2 minutes.
5. Take your egg mixture previously prepared and place it on the warmed up tortillas. Roll the tortillas as you wish and you are ready to enjoy them.

Hibiscus maple mock tail

Ingredients

- ¼ cups of maple syrup
- 8 cups of water
- 2 inches ginger (Grated)
- 2 limes (Juice)
- ½ cup rose petals (Dried)
- 1/3 cup of hibiscus flower (Dried)

Method
1. Take a pot of your choice for boiling. Place water in the pot over medium flame.
2. In the boiling water, add the maple syrup and the grated ginger.
3. After a minute or so, reduce the heat of the flame and simmer the water with the other ingredients for 15 minutes.
4. Simmer for 5 more minutes. When it has simmered enough, add the dried hibiscus flowers and rose petals to the mixture and simmer it for another 5 minutes.
5. When it is done, pour the water through a sieve into a pitcher. Using a sieve will ensure that the petals and ginger will be removed.
6. When the mixture has cooled down, add the lime juice to it and serve.

Papaya Smoothie

Ingredients
- 90 g of papaya (Cut in small pieces)
- 1 teaspoon honey
- ½ cup almond or oat milk (Unsweetened)
- ½ teaspoon fresh ginger, grated
- 2 ice cubes
- 2 tablespoons lime juice

Method

1 Take your blender and add the milk, papaya, ginger, lime and honey to it. Blend them together for 15 seconds.

2 Pour in the ice cubes in the blender. Blend the mixture for about 30 seconds or longer if you feel that it hasn't become smooth yet.

3 You are ready to serve.

Cheerful cherry

Ingredients
- ½ cup orange juice
- ¼ cup tart cherry juice (Unsweetened)
- ¼ cup (about 2) lime juice, freshly squeezed
- 225 ml can club soda
- 2 lime slices (Garnish)

Method

1 Add all the juices in a large glass jar and mix them well. Cover the jar with a lid and put it inside the refrigerator.

2 When you are going to serve, take it out of the refrigerator and uncover the lid.

3 Pour the juice into glasses of your choice or attractive cocktail glasses and top it off with club soda. Garnish with slices of lime or orange, according to your choice and you are ready to serve.

Strawberry cream cheese smoothie

Ingredients
- 1 cup strawberries (Hulled)
- 1 cup rice milk (Unsweetened)
- 2 tablespoons cream cheese, at room temperature
- 1 teaspoon vanilla extract
- ½ teaspoon honey
- 3 to 5 ice cubes

Method

1 Take out your blender and add the rice milk, cream cheese, strawberries, vanilla, honey and ice cubes. Make sure to mix them well. Blend the ingredients until the mixture is smooth and you are ready to serve.

Summer fresh watermelon smoothie

Ingredients
- 4 Cups watermelon (Cubed)
- 2 Limes
- 2 Cups of strawberries
- 6 Large basil leaves
- 2 Cups ice

Method
1. Pour in your strawberries, watermelon and lime juice into your blender.
2. Pour in your ice next. Blend the mixture until it is smooth for about 30 seconds to 1 minute.
3. Choose the glasses that you want to serve in or in individual glasses and garnish it with strawberry slices and basil leaves.

Spiced tea

Ingredients
- 2 Cinnamon sticks
- 5 Cups of water
- 1 piece of turmeric (about 2 inch, peeled and sliced)
- 1 piece of ginger (about 2 inch, peeled and sliced)
- 5 Black peppercorns

1 Take a saucepan or pot and pour in the water. Set the flame to medium.

2 You will need to add the spices next and bring the water to boil.

3 When the water starts boiling, reduce the flame and simmer it for about 30 minutes. 4 When it has been simmered right, pour it into glasses and serve it hot.

Chocolate smoothie

Ingredients
- 2 Cups of ice
- 2 Scoops of chocolate flavoured whey protein
- ½ cup evaporated milk
- ¼ cup condensed milk
- 2 tablespoons of southern comfort liqueur (optional)
- ¼ teaspoon ground cinnamon
- Pinch of nutmeg

Method

1 Take your blender and add all the ingredients to it, except for cinnamon. Mix them nicely. Blend the ingredients at high speed for about 1-2 minutes until the mixture becomes smooth.

2 Take glasses and pour in the mixture and add whipped cream topping. Sprinkle cinnamon as your garnish.

Mixed Berry smoothie in a bowl

Ingredients
- 1 cup mixed frozen berries (Unsweetened)
- 1 packet of frozen acai (Unsweetened)
- 3/4 cup plain 2% low fat Greek yogurt
- 2 tablespoons raspberries
- 1/2 cup rice milk (Unsweetened, original, classic)
- 1 teaspoon chia seeds
- ¼ of a fresh pear
- 2 tablespoons blueberries

Method

1 Take out the frozen acai from the packet and break it up into little pieces.

2 Take your blender and add the acai pieces, Greek yogurt, mixed frozen berries, rice milk and chia seeds. Blend the ingredients until smooth. You will have to make sure that the mixture is thick enough to be eaten with a spoon.

3 Take out two bowls and pour the mixture evenly into them.

4 Top and garnish it with fresh pear pieces, raspberries and blueberries.

Apple Maple granola

Ingredients

- 3 Cups old fashioned oats
- 3 Cups puffed rice cereal
- 100 g package baked apple chips
- 1 and ½ teaspoon ground cinnamon
- ½ cup dried cranberries (sweetened)
- 1 teaspoon ground nutmeg
- 1/4 cup 100% pure maple syrup
- 1/4 cup melted coconut oil
- 1-1/2 teaspoons vanilla extract
- 1/2 cup unsweetened applesauce

Method

1. Turn on your oven and preheat it 135 degree Celsius or 275 degree Fahrenheit. Take two large baking sheets and line them with parchment paper.
2. Take all the dry ingredients in one bowl and mix them well.
3. Take all the wet ingredients in another bowl and make sure to mix them well.
4. Take the wet ingredients bowl and pour everything in the dry ingredients bowl. Make sure to mix them well so that the dry ingredients are coated perfectly.
5. Take your baking sheets and divide the mixture equally on them.
6. You will have to bake the mixture for about 50 minutes to 1 hour. Change the position of the tray half way through baking. Place the bottom tray on top and vice versa.

Scottish blueberry smoothie

Ingredients
- 8 Packets of Splenda
- 1 cup frozen blueberries
- 8 ice cubes
- 6 Tablespoons of protein powder
- 400 ml of apple juice (No added sugar)

Method

1. Place all ingredients in a blender and blend until smooth. Take your blender and add all the ingredients listed above to the blender. Blend the mixture until smooth.
2. Take your preferred glasses and serve the smoothie chilled. You can garnish it with chopped blueberries.

Red carpet Apple juice

Ingredients
- 1/2 medium beet
- 1/2 medium apple
- ¼ cup parsley
- 1 celery stalk
- 1 medium fresh carrot

1. Take your juicer and add your beet, carrot, apple and parsley to it. You will need to extract

the juice from the ingredients.
2. Take two small glasses of your choice and pour the drink into it. You can drink it right away
or put in the refrigerator to cool.

Protein Berry Shake

Ingredients
- 1/2 cup sherbet
- 1/4 cup low-cholesterol egg product
- 1/2 cup soy milk
- 3 tablespoons whey protein powder
- 1/4 cup cranberry juice
- 1/2 cup frozen blueberries
- 2 ice cubes

Method
1 Blend ingredients in a blender for 30 to 45 seconds.
2 Divide into two servings. Serve one now; freeze the second serving for later.

Stir fried breakfast chicken

Ingredients
- 360g chicken breast (Boneless and skinless)
- 3 Tablespoons honey
- 3 Tablespoons vinegar
- 3 Tablespoons pineapple juice
- 1 and a 1/2 tablespoon reduced-sodium soy sauce
- 1 and a 1/2 teaspoon cornstarch
- 2 Tablespoons canola oil
- 3 Cups frozen mixed vegetables
- 3 Cups hot cooked rice

Method
1 Rinse chicken; pat dry. Cut chicken into 1-inch pieces; set aside.

2 To make sauce, stir together honey, vinegar, pineapple juice, soy sauce, and cornstarch; set aside.

3 Pour canola oil into a large skillet or wok. (Add more oil as necessary during cooking.) Preheat over medium high heat.

4 Stir-fry frozen vegetables for 3 minutes or until vegetables are crisp-tender.

5 Remove vegetables from skillet.

6 Add chicken to hot skillet. Stir-fry for 3-4 minutes or until chicken is no longer pink. Push chicken away from the center of the skillet. Stir sauce; add to center of the skillet. Cook and stir until thickened and bubbly.

7 Return cooked vegetables to skillet. Stir all ingredients together to coat. Cook and stir about 1 minute more or until heated through.

8 Serve immediately over rice.

Watermelon coolie

Ingredients
- 1 cup crushed ice
- 1 cup seedless watermelon cubes
- 2 teaspoons lime juice
- 1 tablespoon sugar
- 2 small watermelon wedges for garnish

Method
1. Place all ingredients except garnish wedges in a blender and blend for 30 seconds.
2. Pour into 2 small glasses, garnish with wedges and enjoy!

Raspberry sorbet

Ingredients
- 4 litre canned pineapple juice
- 180ml frozen pink lemonade concentrate
- 480ml raspberry sherbet or sorbet
- 2 liters diet ginger ale (Chilled)
- 300g frozen red raspberries (Thawed)

Method
1. In a large punch bowl, mix together juice, lemonade, sherbet or sorbet and diet ginger ale.
2. Stir in un-drained, thawed raspberries.

Lemon coolie

Ingredients
- 4 Large ice cubes
- 1 tablespoon lemon juice
- 1/4 cup half & half creamer
- 3 Tablespoons sugar

Method
1. Place all ingredients in a blender.
2. Set on ice/crush setting and blend for 30 seconds to one minute or until ice is well chopped and slush is at desired consistency.
3. Pour into a glass and garnish with lemon wedge, if desired.

Lemonade slushie

Ingredients
- 1/3 cup fresh lemon juice
- 1/2 cup strawberries (Fresh) (Unsweetened/Frozen)
- 1 tablespoon sugar or preferred sweetener
- 1/2 cup ice cubes

Method

1. In a blender combine strawberries, lemon juice, and 1 tablespoon sugar or Splenda. Blend until smooth.
2. With blender running, add 1/2 cup ice cubes, one at a time, through opening in lid until beverage is slushy.
3. Sip slowly to enjoy.

Renal Diet Chicken Tikka

Ingredients

- 3 Tablespoons Yogurt (low fat)
- 1 tablespoon Curry paste
- 1 teaspoon Lemon juice
- 2 Boneless Chicken breasts (without skin)
- 1 teaspoon olive oil
- Fresh lettuce for garnish (shredded)
- Salt to taste (low sodium)

Method

1. Take a mixing bowl and mix yogurt and curry paste.
2. Put the chicken in the yogurt mixture and add lemon juice and salt.
3. Let it sit for an hour or marinate it in a refrigerator overnight for best infusion of flavor in the meat.
4. Preheat the grill and brush some olive oil.
5. Cook the chicken on the grill for 15 minutes turning the chicken periodically.
6. Remove the chicken from the grill when cooked properly keeping its juice intact.
7. Serve hot with fresh shredded lettuce or with tortilla wrap for

having it as a snack or served with boiled rice and have it as a main meal.

Renal Diet salad (Kidney beans and sweet corn)

Ingredients

- 450g sweet corn (canned)
- 450g kidney beans (canned)
- 100 g feta cheese (crumbled)
- ½ of a cucumber (finely diced)
- 30 g fresh coriander leaves (finely chopped)
- 60 g fresh parsley (chopped)
- 1 spring onion (finely chopped)
- ½ tablespoon lime juice (for dressing)
- 2 tablespoon olive oil (for dressing)
- 1 teaspoon mustard (for dressing)
- 1 teaspoon cumin (for dressing)
- ½ teaspoon dried oregano (for dressing)
- 1 teaspoon honey (for dressing)
- Salt to taste (low sodium)
- Black Pepper powder to taste

Method

1. Take the canned corn and kidney beans and wash them thoroughly. Place them onto a perforated bowl or plate to help the water to seep out.
2. Take the cucumber and remove the seeds from it. Dice the cucumber nicely.
3. Take coriander leaves and parsley and chop them up into fine pieces.
4. Wash the spring onions and take the green portions and chop them up finely.
5. Take a big bowl to mix everything.
6. Take the sweet corn, kidney beans, diced cucumber, parsley and coriander leaves that has been chopped along with the chopped spring onions. Add all these to the bowl.
7. Crumble the feta cheese and also add it to the mixture in the bowl.
8. You will need a separate bowl for all the dressing ingredients. Take them together and mix them well.
9. Taste both the salad and the dressing to make sure that the seasoning is on point.
10. If you find that the dressing is perfect for your tastes, mix it with the salad.
11. Take chopped coriander leaves and garnish the salad and you are ready to serve.

Oats Granola

Ingredients

- 2 tablespoons of honey
- 4 tablespoons of sunflower oil
- 2 tablespoons of brown sugar
- 1 tablespoon of lemon juice
- 300 g rolled oats
- Dried cranberries (for Garnish)

Method

1. Turn on your oven and preheat it to 280-degree Fahrenheit or 140-degree Celsius.
2. In a large saucepan, take some oil. Add lemon juice, honey and sugar. You will have to heat it on a very low flame so that all the ingredients are perfectly melted and mixed. When everything is melted, add in the oats and mix it in.
3. You will need a baking tray to pour in the ingredients from the saucepan and tilt it or use a spatula to spread it out evenly on the tray.
4. Take this tray and put it inside the oven and bake for around 30-40 minutes until you see the mixture has become crisp. You will need to check granola that is being baked at regular intervals to make sure it is being evenly baked.
5. After it is done, remove the tray from the oven and let it cool down.
6. You can garnish your granola with dried cranberries and serve it or you have the option of storing it in air tight containers for up to 1 month.

Minted Lamb Chops

Ingredients

- 100 g breadcrumbs (homemade or shop brought)
- 1 tablespoon of fresh mint
- 1 tablespoon of fresh parsley
- 2 Lamb chops
- 100 g flour
- 1 free-range egg, whisked
- 1 tbsp. of vegetable or olive oil

Methods

1. Take a blender and add mint, bread crumbs and parsley. Blend them together until they are well combined. Take them out in a bowl.
2. Take your lamb chops and coat them in flour first. Dip them into eggs and then finally into the breadcrumbs and they are well coated with all the ingredients. Season them with pepper.
3. Take a frying pan and heat oil at medium flame. Place the coated lamb chops into the frying pan and cook for three minutes.
4. When one side is done, turn it over and cook for another three minutes until both sides are done nicely.
5. Take out the chops from the frying pan and place them on a plate. Let them rest for about three minutes and you are ready to serve.

Grilled corn on the cob

Ingredients

- Corn on the cob (Husks on)
- Margarine
- Pepper to taste
- 4 square of aluminium foil (Large enough to wrap individual corn on the cobs)

Method

1 Take out your outdoor grill and preheat it at high, 400 degree Fahrenheit or 205 degree Celsius.

2 You will have to remove the corn husks and the silk or the hair on the corn by peeling it carefully.

3 Rub margarine and pepper on all the sides of the corn. Make sure to rub everywhere. Take the husks and close them around the corn.

4 Wrap the aluminium tightly around each ear of corn. You will have to make sure to seal the edges tightly so that there is no leakage. When you are done, place the corn on the preheated grill.

5 You will have to cook the corn until it has become tender, for about 25-30 minutes approximately. Keep turning it to different sides so that it doesn't burn.

Turkey and pasta salad

Ingredients

- 3 Cups of pasta (Elbow or shell or bowtie)
- 470 g cooked turkey breast (Unsalted, cubed)
- ¼ cup chopped celery
- 2 Tablespoon Carrot (Shredded)
- 2 Tablespoons Red bell pepper (Chopped)
- 2 Tablespoons Purple onion (Finely chopped)
- ½ cup mayonnaise
- 1/8 tsp. Pepper
- 1 tbsp. Lemon juice
- ½ tsp. Sugar

Method

1. Take a bowl and add the pasta, red bell pepper, turkey, celery, purple onion and carrot. Mix all of them together nicely.
2. Take your blender and add mayonnaise, pepper, lemon juice and sugar. Blend all of them together nicely and it has become smooth. Take out another bowl to take it out.
3. Now you are ready to pour the dressing into your vegetable and turkey salad that you have already prepared. Make sure to have all of it well coated with the dressing. Chill the salad mixture and you are ready to serve.

Gardener's chicken and berry salad

Ingredients

- 1/3 cup celery (Chopped)
- cups of chicken (Diced)
- ¼ cup fresh onion (Chopped)
- 1 teaspoon dry mustard
- 1 teaspoon parsley (Dried) (optional)
- ¼ teaspoon black pepper
- 1 tablespoon lemon juice
- ¼ cup fresh green pepper (Chopped)
- ½ cup mayonnaise

Method

1. Take a bowl and add onion, chicken, celery, parsley, green pepper and mix it with lemon juice.
2. Take another bowl and add mustard, black pepper and mayonnaise. Mix them together to make the sauce and then add it to the bowl of chicken mixture. Coat the chicken nicely with the sauce.

Stir fry delight

Ingredients

- 2 Cups of cooked rice
- ½ tablespoon soy sauce (low sodium)
- 1 packet of stir fry vegetables (frozen, 100 g)
- 2 Chicken breasts (medium size, cut into bite size pieces)
- 2 Tablespoons cooking oil

Method

1. Take a 9 inch or 10 inch skillet and heat oil in it.
2. Add chicken, and sauté. Add the chicken and sauté it in the skillet. Then add the vegetables to the chicken.
3. Add the soy sauce now and stir well, mixing everything thoroughly.
4. Take down the flame to medium and cook the vegetables and chicken for 3-5 minutes or until you feel that the food is done. Keep stirring the food constantly.
5. You ready to serve the food with 2/3 cups of rice.

Barbecue muffins

Ingredients

- ½ cup spicy barbecue sauce (Low sodium)
- ¾ pounds of lean turkey (Grounded)
- 2 Teaspoons onion flakes
- 300 g of refrigerator biscuits (Low fat, 1 packet)
- Dash of garlic powder

Method

1. Take oil in a pan or a skillet. Add the ground turkey meat to it and cook it until you see it turning brown.

2. Now as the turkey has browned, add the barbecue sauce along with garlic powder and onion flakes. Make sure to mix them well.

3. Take a muffin tin and flatten each biscuit to the bottom of the tin.

4. Take a spoon and place enough of the turkey mixture to the centre of each of the biscuits.

5. Bake the muffins at 400 degree Fahrenheit or 205 degree Celsius for about 10 to 12 minutes.

6. Plate the muffins when the time is up and they are baked perfectly. You are ready to serve.

Crusty crackers patty

Ingredients

- 1 egg (egg substitute or egg white optional)

- ⅓ Cup low sodium crackers
- 1/3 cup green or red peppers (Finely chopped)
- 1 tablespoon dry mustard
- ¼ cup mayonnaise (Reduced fat)
- 1 teaspoon crushed red pepper or black pepper
- 2 tablespoons vegetable oil
- 1 teaspoon garlic powder
- 2 tablespoons lemon juice

Method

1. Take a bowl and add all the ingredients together. Mix them well.
2. Divide the mixture into 6 balls and pat them with your hand to make patties.
3. Take some vegetable oil in a pan or skillet and heat it at medium flame or you can use your oven to make the patties. Heat the oven at 175 degree Celsius or 350 degree Fahrenheit.
4. You can fry the patties for 4-5 minutes in the oil or you can bake it in the oven for 15 minutes. Serve the patties warm.

Shrimp salad

Ingredients

- 1 hardboiled egg (Chopped)
- 1 pound of shrimp (Boiled, chopped, deveined)
- 1 tablespoon celery (Chopped)
- 1 tablespoon onion (Chopped)
- 1 tablespoon green pepper(Chopped)
- 2 tablespoons mayonnaise
- ½ teaspoon chilli powder
- 1 teaspoon lemon juice
- ⅛ Teaspoon Tabasco or hot sauce
- ½ teaspoon dry mustard
- Lettuce (Chopped or shredded) (optional)

Method

1. Take a bowl and mix all the ingredients together, leaving out the lettuce.
2. Put the mixture in the refrigerator for 30 minutes.
3. You have the option of serving it on wraps of lettuce or you can serve it on sandwich.

www.ingramcontent.com/pod-product-compliance
Lightning Source LLC
Chambersburg PA
CBHW080623030426
42336CB00018B/3054